SECOND EDITION

HEALTHY SHOULDER HANDBOOK

100 EXERCISES

FOR TREATING COMMON INJURIES AND ENDING CHRONIC PAIN

DR. KARL KNOPF

ULYSSES PRESS

Published in the US by:
Ulysses Press
PO Box 3440
Berkeley, CA 94703
www.ulyssespress.com

ISBN: 978-1-64604-196-1
Library of Congress Control Number: 2021931498

Printed in Canada by Marquis Book Printing
10 9 8 7 6 5 4 3 2 1

Contributing writer: Fiona Gilbert
Acquisitions: Claire Seilaff
Managing editor: Claire Chun
Editor: Renee Rutledge
Proofreader: Barbara Schultz
Index: Sayre Van Young
Front cover design: Rebecca Lown
Interior design: what!design @ whatweb.com
Artwork: cover illustration © autumnn/shutterstock.com; illustrations on pages 7 and 9 © angelhell/istockphoto.com; photographs © Rapt Productions
Production: Jake Flaherty
Models: Samuel Harvell, Scott Mathison, Meredith Miller, Bernadett Otterbein, Toni Silver

PLEASE NOTE: This book has been written and published strictly for informational purposes, and in no way should be used as a substitute for consultation with health care professionals. You should not consider educational material herein to be the practice of medicine or to replace consultation with a physician or other medical practitioner. The author and publisher are providing you with information in this work so that you can have the knowledge and can choose, at your own risk, to act on that knowledge. The author and publisher also urge all readers to be aware of their health status and to consult health care professionals before beginning any health program.

CONTENTS

PART 1: GETTING STARTED 1

INTRODUCTION 2

Who Gets Shoulder Issues? . . . . 3 Do I Have a Shoulder Issue? 4

SHOULDER ANATOMY 6

Bones and Joints . . . . 6 The Joint Capsule 8
The Supporting Cast . . . . 7 Muscles 8

COMMON SHOULDER CONDITIONS 10

Shoulder Impingement . . . . 11 Rotator Cuff Injuries 16
Repetitive Motion Injuries . . . . 12 Frozen Shoulder 17
Shoulder Instability   Tendinitis and Bursitis 18
(Dislocation/Subluxation) . . . . 14 Thoracic Outlet Syndrome (TOS) 20
Arthritis 15

SHOULDER REHAB 24

Injury Classifications . . . . 25 The Healing Process 25

PART 2: PREVENTIVE AND SPECIALIZED PROGRAMS 29

PREVENTING (RE)INJURY 30

Posture's Role in Prevention . . . . 32 The Green, Yellow, and Red Zones 33

CONTROVERSIAL EXERCISES 36

DESIGNING A SHOULDER ROUTINE 40

Sample Conditioning Programs . . . . .43 Swimming 47
General Conditioning . . . . .44 Tennis 47
Baseball/Softball . . . . .44 Volleyball .48
Basketball .45 Wrestling or Mixed Martial Arts 48
Football . . . . .45 Construction Job 49
Golf . . . . .46 Office/Desk Job 49
Hockey 46

SPECIALIZED CORRECTIVE EXERCISE PROGRAMS 50

Shoulder Impingement. 51
Repetitive Injury Series 51
Rotator Cuff Injuries 51

Tendinitis and Bursitis. 52
Shoulder Dislocations. 52
Frozen Shoulder 52

PART 3: SHOULDER CONDITIONING EXERCISES 53

THE EXERCISES 54

Passive & Gentle Series 55
Pendulum (Forward and Backward). 55
Pendulum (Across Body). 56
Hanging Arm Circles 57
Shoulder Box 58
Shoulder Rolls 59
Elbow Touches. 60
Pec Stretch 61
Apple Pickers. 62
Picture Frame 63
Table Reach 64
Choker 65
Over the Top 66
Internal Rotation Stretch. 67
Arm Pulls 68
Table Stretch 69

Active Range of Motion Series 70
Angels. 70
Soup Can Pours 71
Upper-Back Stretch. 72
The Wave 73
Shoulder Blade Pinch 74
Wood Chops 75
Condor. 76
Rescue Me 77
Touch Down 78

Push Backs. 79
The Zipper 80
Rotator Cuff (External Rotation) 81

Floor Series 82
Elbow Touches (Supine). 82
Finger Circles 83
Straight-Arm Stretch. 84
I's, Y's, and T's 85
Crossing Guard 87
External Rotation (Supine) 88
Internal Rotation (Supine) 89
Internal Rotation (Side-Lying) 90
External Rotation (Side-Lying). 91
Shoulder Blade Push-Up 92

Cane/Stick Series 93
Supine Press 93
Pull-Overs 94
Lateral Drops 95
Reverse Lift 96
Stick Press 97
Back Scratch 98

Roller Series 99
Windmills on Roller 100
Elbow Drops 101
Shoulder Slaps. 102
I's, Y's, and T's on Roller. 103

Wall/Door Series **105**
Finger Walking (Forward) 105
Finger Walking (Side) 106
Side Clock 107
Wall Circles .108
Corner Stretch 109
Chest Stretch (Doorway) 110
Stick Up 111
Elbow Touches (Against Wall) 112
Double-Hand Press 113
Wall Reach 114
External Rotation (Wall) 115
Internal Rotation (Door) 116
Wall Push-Up 117
Isometric Shoulder Blade Squeeze 118
Isometric Frontal Lift 119
Isometric Rear Lift 120
Static Pec Stretch 121

Resistance Conditioning Series **122**
Frontal Raises 123
Lateral Raises 124
Shoulder Extension 125
Reverse Fly with Band 126
Downward Sword Fighter 127
Sword Fighter 128
Bike Pump 129
Horizontal Triceps Extension 130
Serving Tray 131
Internal Rotation with Band 132

External Rotation with Band 133
Seated Rowing 134
Pull-Downs 135
Band Chest Press 136
Band Shoulder Press 137
Y's with Band 138
T's with Band 139
Band Roll-Ups .140
Shrug 141

Dumbbell Series **142**
Dumbbell Shoulder Extension 142
Dumbbell Soup Can Pours 143
Dumbbell Reverse Fly 144
Dumbbell Press-Up 145
Dumbbell Shrugs 146
Hanging Dumbbell Squeeze 147
Prone Crossing Guard 148

Self-Massage **149**
Tennis Ball Method 1 149
Tennis Ball Method 2 150
Tennis Ball Method 3 150
Tennis Ball Method 4 151
Tennis Ball Method 5 151
Tennis Ball Method 6 152
Tennis Ball Method 7 152
Foam Roller (Back) 153
Foam Roller (Side) 154
Ice 155

RESOURCES 156

INDEX 157

ACKNOWLEDGMENTS 162

ABOUT THE AUTHOR 162

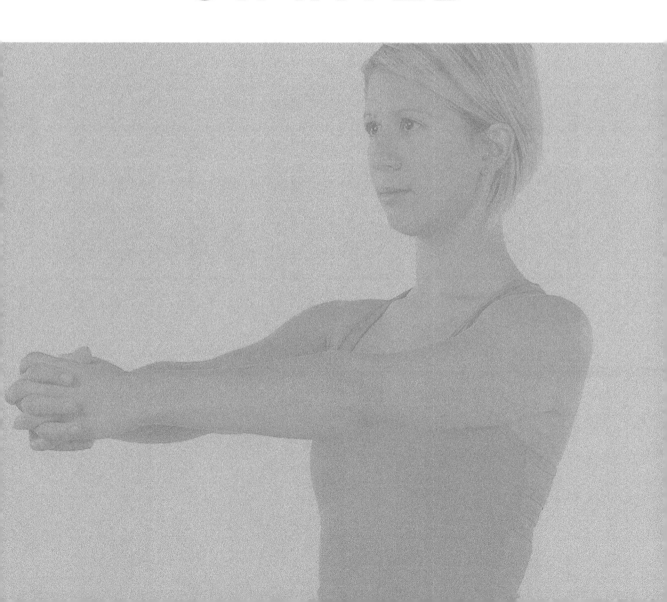

PART 1

GETTING
STARTED

INTRODUCTION

This book provides an overview of shoulder anatomy, as well as common causes of injuries to better understand prevention. The goal of this book is to acquaint you with possible shoulder conditions and offer suggestions for prevention and corrective exercise options. Many physical therapy textbooks and journals were reviewed to make sure the information contained within is credible and has scientific background. However, this is by no means a substitute for medical care. The hope of this book is for you to learn to TRAIN SMART, NOT HARD, because learning to listen to your body and heed what it says is the wisest thing you can do. Identifying a small shoulder issue and engaging in active rest along with performing corrective exercise can go a long way in keeping you in the game.

With the supervision of a doctor, anyone can use this book to strengthen an injured shoulder or identify the onset of a shoulder problem.

The shoulder joint is complex, remarkable, and subject to injury. Shoulder dysfunction is caused by many variables: falls, overuse, misuse, and even disuse after an injury. Shoulder mobility can also be impaired after cancer treatments. Injury to the soft tissue surrounding the shoulder joint may very well be prevented if you engage in a proactive, progressive strengthening and stretching program of corrective exercises.

Often the onset of a shoulder problem manifests slowly over time and if neglected, it impairs function or causes excessive pain. Shoulder pain is reported to occur in 20 percent of the adult population. Too often, people hurt or strain their shoulder and dismiss the injury, only to allow it to exacerbate to a significant issue. The current belief is getting therapy and treatment early can prevent major problems in the future. Being proactive about the care of your shoulder as a preventive method now, before something big happens, is the best idea.

The good news is most people with shoulder pain can both improve function and reduce pain through physical therapy and corrective exercise. According to the *Journal of Orthopaedic & Sports Physical Therapy*, shoulder exercises are an excellent way to manage pain and improve function.

WHO GETS SHOULDER ISSUES?

Statistics show that a significant number of the adult population has or will suffer from a shoulder joint dysfunction that affects daily activities. A shoulder dysfunction is no small problem; it can disable you for a sustained period of time.

Other than trauma and repetitive chronic misuses, often postural deviations or muscle imbalances can contribute to shoulder issues. If one set of muscles gets too tight, the delicate balance of the space in the shoulder complex is upset, possibly throwing the alignment out of place. This is similar to the guide wires of a radio tower; if they're too tight, they can cause misalignment. These misalignments set the stage for injury. With proper joint alignment, you can expect an ideal range of motion. (Perhaps if we follow Joseph Pilates's advice of strengthening what is weak and stretching what is tight, some of our shoulder issues will never occur.)

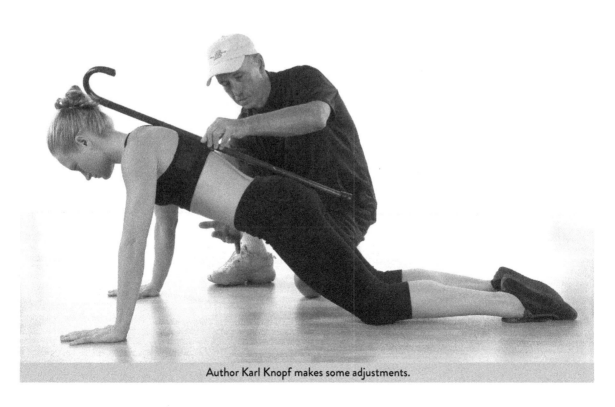

Author Karl Knopf makes some adjustments.

According to the American Academy of Orthopedic Surgeons, shoulder dysfunction is caused by many situations, including falls and overuse from work or play. Today we even see children complaining of shoulder and neck pain caused by poor posture, poor biomechanics while playing computer games, back and shoulder strain from carrying heavy backpacks, or overzealous coaches pushing them beyond their physical limits.

The most common causes of shoulder issues include:

- Age
- Falls
- Improper body mechanics
- Repetitive or prolonged overhead movements
- Prolonged use of machinery that causes jarring/vibration of shoulder joint

DO I HAVE A SHOULDER ISSUE?

Unfortunately, many people wait too long before going to the doctor about their shoulder problem, assuming it will just get better on its own. Research suggests that most people don't go to the doctor until they've lost some level of range of motion or the pain is unbearable. Proactive steps such as medical care and gentle movement are the keys to recovering from shoulder issues.

Ironically, the natural response to stop using the shoulder when it hurts may actually contribute to a condition called "frozen shoulder."

If you suspect that you have a shoulder issue, get a diagnosis ASAP. An early intervention can keep a small issue from becoming a big one. Make an appointment with your primary care doctor, who's usually the port of entry into the medical system. Your primary care doctor may then refer you to other health professionals.

If you have pain or difficulty with any of the following, it's a sign that you may have a shoulder problem and should seek medical advice.

- Putting on a coat
- Sleeping on your side
- Reaching behind you, as when grabbing something in the backseat of the car from the driver's seat)
- Reaching up your back, as when zipping up a back zipper
- Reaching to a high shelf
- Throwing a ball overhand
- Performing work duties, such as moving a computer mouse around on the desk

- Participating in recreational pursuits, such as swimming the crawl stroke or playing tennis

If you have any of the above or hear a pop, get a diagnosis ASAP.

WHAT TO EXPECT WHEN YOU VISIT YOUR DOCTOR

Be prepared to:

- Explain your functional limitations.
- Explain when it hurts and where. Be specific.
- Explain how much it hurts on a scale of 1 to 10.

The health professional may:

- Take X-rays.
- Refer you to physical therapy.
- Prescribe rest or medication or an injection.

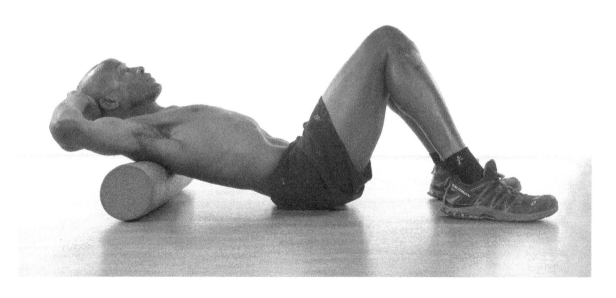

SHOULDER ANATOMY

BONES AND JOINTS

The shoulder girdle is composed of four bones:

- The **clavicle** is commonly known as the collar bone.
- The **scapula** is also known as the shoulder blades, or wing/angel bones; the *acromion* is the part of the scapula that forms a bony roof above the rotator cuff, tendons, and bursa.
- The **sternum** is often referred to as the breastbone.
- The **humerus** is the upper bone of the arm.

Joints, where bones come together, are surrounded by soft tissue, which includes ligaments, tendons, and bursas. There are several joints/articulations of the shoulder. The majority of the joint movement occurs in the GH joint; the other joints serve more as supporting structures.

- **Acromioclavicular (AC)**—This joint is formed by the acromion and the clavicle. Mainly, it is active with shrugging movements.
- **Glenohumeral (GH)**—The combination of the upper arm bone and the outside area of the scapula makes up this joint. This joint is responsible for most of the movements of the shoulder. Shoulder dislocation always refers to this joint.
- **Sternoclavicular (SC)**—This joint is composed of the clavicle and the sternum. This joint primarily operates during shrugs, although part of its function is to stabilize the shoulder girdle.
- **Scapulothoracic (ST)**—This is not really a movable joint but serves as a base for muscles to be secured to.

THE SUPPORTING CAST

LIGAMENTS AND TENDONS

Ligaments are fibrous connective tissue that attach bone to bone. It is also known as articular ligament, fibrous ligament, or true ligament. Often, with age, ligaments lose tensile strength, setting up the potential for injury. The ligaments of the shoulder region are the acromioclavicular ligament, also known as the AC joint ligament, and the coracoclavicular ligament.

A tendon is a tough band of fibrous connective tissue that connects muscle to bone and is capable of withstanding tension. Tendons are similar to ligaments; both are made of collagen.

The shoulder joint's ligaments and tendons keep it stable, but these bands can become lax through misuse and chronic overuse. Each type of fiber has a unique role to play and offers different abilities. The complexity of the shoulder joint allows it to be one of the most mobile joints of the body. This mobility, however, is also why the shoulder joint is so vulnerable to overuse and injuries, and one reason why it's the most difficult and complicated joint in the body to rehabilitate.

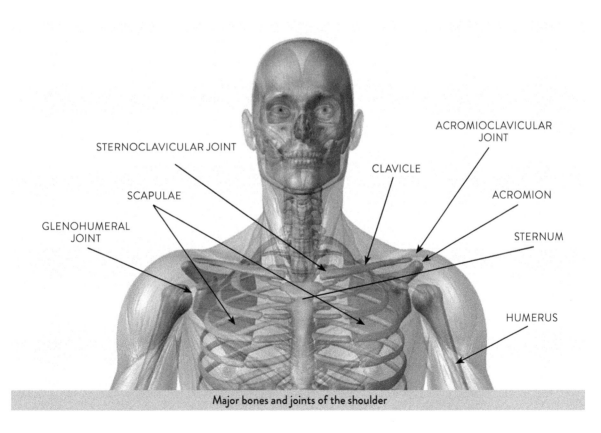

Major bones and joints of the shoulder

Each of the four rotary cuff muscles originates on the scapula, and their tendons attach to the top of the humerus, helping to form the joint capsule. The sac surrounding the joint is called a bursa. A fluid-filled bursa is usually found between bones and tendons to help decrease friction during normal joint use. It provides lubrication to the joint.

THE JOINT CAPSULE

CARTILAGE

Cartilage is the gristle/pad between joints, providing cushion. The cartilage is designed to provide a smooth surface for joint bones to glide over. Often, with use, these once-smooth surfaces wear down. Once they break down, as seen in osteoarthritis, pain and inflammation (redness, soreness, swelling) occur.

BURSA

The sac surrounding the joint is called a bursa. A fluid-filled bursa is usually found between bones and tendons to help decrease friction during normal joint use. It provides lubrication to the joint. Many times, after frequent insults and impingements, the bursa becomes inflamed, causing pain that can lead to restricted movement.

MUSCLES

Before we move on to the muscles of the shoulder, remember that muscles can do two things: contract or relax. Agonist muscles are responsible for contraction movements, while antagonist muscles produce an action opposite of the agonist. In addition, stabilizer muscles anchor or support a bone so the agonist can have a firm base from which to operate (the rotator cuff muscles are a good example of a stabilizer muscle).

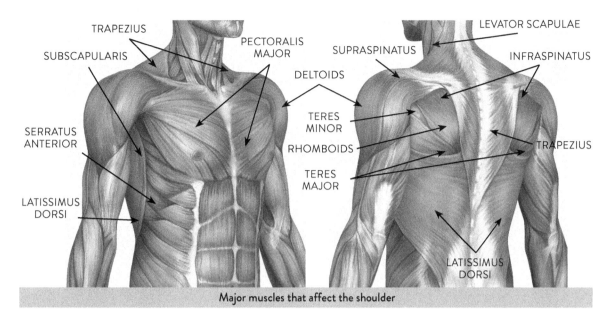

Major muscles that affect the shoulder

The major muscles of the shoulder region are sometimes broken down into either stabilizers or dynamic muscles of the joint. The muscles below serve to influence the motions available at the shoulder joint.

Static stabilizers:

- **Supraspinatus** abducts the arm (i.e., moves the arm away from the body).
- **Infraspinatus** rotates the arm laterally.
- **Teres minor** rotates the arm laterally.
- **Teres major** adducts the arm (i.e., brings the arm into the body).
- **Subscapularis** internally rotates the arm.

Dynamic stabilizers (prime movers):

- **Latissimus dorsi** extends and adducts the arm.
- **Trapezius** elevates and depresses the scapula.
- **Pectoralis major and minor** adduct the arm and pull the scapula downward.
- **Coracobrachialis** flexes and adducts the arm.
- **Deltoid** abducts and extends the arm.
- **Levator scapulae** moves the neck laterally.
- **Rhomboid major and minor** stabilize the scapula.
- **Serratus anterior** stabilizes the scapula.

COMMON SHOULDER CONDITIONS

As with most joint conditions, shoulder problems can be traced back to misuse, overuse, disuse or abuse of shoulder muscles. Anything that affects any part of the kinetic chain can cause problems. For instance, taking a bad fall (abuse) or painting the ceiling for two hours straight (misuse/overuse) may result in an unhappy shoulder.

Other factors contributing to shoulder dysfunctions include neurology, physiological variants, and age.

Neurology. In order for muscles to function properly, the neuropathway from the muscles to the brain must be functional. Several pathways innervate the muscles of the shoulder region, and any dysfunction or disruption to those neuropathways will limit both motor and feeling functions. An injury to the brain, therefore, may contribute to dysfunction.

Physiological variants. In order for the shoulder joint to function properly, the tendons that attach the muscles must be intact. When this variant is impaired you will hear terms like "tendinitis."

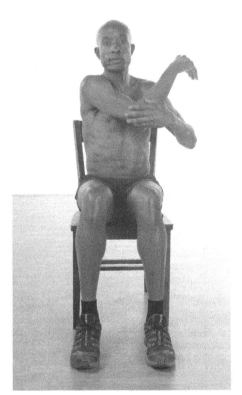

Age. While age alone does not cause shoulder problems, unfortunately, age does play a factor in shoulder conditions. As we age, the soft tissues surrounding the shoulder girdle undergo some structural changes. Often, these structural changes lead to the weakening of the supporting ligaments, tendons, and muscles. Some experts in the field suggest that by 50 years of age, most people have some internal shoulder structural changes. Often, a simple tendinitis can degenerate into actual tearing of the muscle tissues. If simple tendinitis is not properly treated, further episodes can lead to greater damage—which is why early intervention and preventative maintenance is the key to complete shoulder health.

The overview of common shoulder conditions provided in this section includes typical causes, symptoms, and treatments. Unless you're an expert on shoulders, it is always recommended that you consult your doctor, who will take a health history and do a physical exam for an accurate diagnosis.

Your doctor may also perform a highly regarded assessment tool called the subjective shoulder scale assessment, used with rotator cuff, shoulder instability, and arthritis clients. During this assessment, you'll be evaluated on whether you experience difficulty putting on a coat, sleeping on your side, reaching behind you, combing your hair, reaching a high shelf, throwing a ball overhand, or performing work duties or recreational pursuits.

For corrective exercise programs for these conditions, see Specialized Corrective Exercise Programs on page 50.

SHOULDER IMPINGEMENT

Shoulder impingement is a chronic condition sometimes seen in people who are extremely hypermobile. That extra flexibility leads to repetitive stress and inflammation.

Common Symptoms

- Pinching sensation when raising arm
- Pain when sleeping on one side
- Pain accompanying arm movement

Common Causes

Shoulder impingement can be caused by repetitive activity that requires the shoulder joint to do overhead motions day in and day out, such as:

- Tennis
- Swimming

- Throwing sports, such as baseball and softball
- Regular excessive overhead arm motions, such as from working in a warehouse or conducting home repairs
- Sleeping on the same arm each night
- Trauma, such as falling on shoulder

Assessment

- Range-of-motion tests
- A simple assessment of muscle imbalances and muscle testing, during which the health practitioner uses manual resistance to compare the weakness of the affected side against the unaffected side
- X-ray or MRI

Treatment

The doctor may offer you many options, including rest, learning to use your shoulder in a more biomechanically correct fashion, physical therapy modalities, corrective exercises, injections, and surgery. The therapist or doctor may also:

- Instruct you on how to use heat and ice.
- Recommend medication and medicated pads.
- Apply electrical stimulation or ultrasound treatments.
- Suggest steroid injections in the joint area.

REPETITIVE MOTION INJURIES

Anyone who uses the same arm over and over again for either work or recreation is at risk for repetitive motion injuries, also known as cumulative trauma disorder. That is because these repetitive motions can aggravate the shoulder joint structures, such as the tendons, ligaments bursa sac, or cartilage. If unchecked, repetitive motion injuries can lead to further inflammation and decreased range of motion.

Rotator cuff tears are seen quite often in those between the ages of 45 and 65. The most familiar causes for repetitive injuries include overuse with throwing sports and poor execution of exercises in the weight room, such as lat pulls behind the neck or improper bench presses (see page 36 for common controversial exercises). Repetitive motion injuries and trauma often lead to rotator cuff injuries, which are the result of:

- Overuse tendinitis: Leads to irritation and fraying of the tendon.
- Impingement tendinitis: The acromion can pinch and irritate the rotator cuff, or the bursa is swollen as a result of repetitive overhead motion.
- Calcification tendinitis: Inflammation can lead to calcium deposits within the rotator cuff.
- Severe tendinitis: Tears can cause partial or complete tearing of the rotator cuff.

Common Symptoms

- Pain in shoulder, hand, or arm when lying on that side of the body
- Numbness in arm or fingers
- Tingling in hands, arm, or fingers
- Chronic aching in shoulder or arm

Common Causes

- Repetitive overhead motion
- Repetitive use of forceful movement

Assessment

During your assessment, your doctor will take a health history, asking many questions about when your shoulder hurts and how you think you hurt it. Your doctor will perform a physical exam looking for signs of weakness, taking you through a series of movements with and without resistance to evaluate the specific issues you have. The most important thing you can do to expedite the exam is to specify which movements bring the most discomfort. The health practitioner will also ask you if the pain comes on suddenly, and which activities make it worse.

If a diagnosis cannot be made from the physical exam, the doctor may order imaging tests such as MRIs, x-rays, and arthrograms (dye is injected into the shoulder for this procedure).

Treatment

Generally, most doctors will first prescribe a conservative care regimen of rest, cold packs, heat packs, and medication. If that does not work, you may be referred to physical therapy, where corrective exercises along with ultrasound (gentle sound-wave vibrations) and electrical stimulation treatments may be administered. Some doctors will use cortisone injections to reduce the inflammation. If these fail to bring relief, surgical options may be discussed.

SHOULDER INSTABILITY (DISLOCATION/SUBLUXATION)

Due to its design, the shoulder joint is one of the most frequently dislocated joints of the body. The dislocation often results from a strong force that pulls the shoulder/arm outward or through an extreme rotation that "pops" the ball (the head of the humerus) out of the joint. Note that partial dislocations are possible. Since many dislocations come with an associated fracture or nerve damage, they are considered serious. A first-time dislocation is accompanied by intense pain; recurrent dislocations may be less painful.

In a subluxation, the shoulder feels like it slipped out of the socket then slipped back into place. Rather than being a complete dislocation or separation, the head of the humerus slides over the labrum then returns to normal position. Having a complete separation/dislocation is far more damaging and, once a shoulder dislocates, dislocations can occur more frequently.

Common Symptoms

* The arm is physically out of the joint, making it impossible to move. There is also moderate pain.

Common Causes

* Falling
* Running into something/someone
* Lifting incorrectly
* Reaching past your safety zone

Assessment

The health practitioner will look at the joint and see if it's displaced. They will also determine whether or not you're able to move the arm.

Treatment

If you suspect you have any level of separation of the shoulder joint, IMMEDIATELY go to a trained professional to have it repositioned. Once the joint has been repositioned, follow the doctor's orders and an exercise routine to improve the stability of the joint. See the shoulder dislocations corrective exercise program on page 52 for corrective exercises.

ARTHRITIS

Osteoarthritis of the shoulder is a degenerative condition in which the cartilage deteriorates. This is often the result of chronic wear and tear. However, it can be caused by disease, trauma, or infection. Arthritis of the shoulder is seen in the AC joint earlier than the GH joint because the AC joint degenerates more quickly.

POLYMYALGIA RHEUMATICA

This is an inflammatory condition causing pain in the morning and stiffness in the shoulders, neck, and hips. It affects mostly women over 50. This condition should be overseen by a physical therapist and rheumatologist for proper treatment.

Common Symptoms

- Mild to moderate pain in the shoulder area
- Limited range of motion

Common Causes

- Wear and tear
- Rheumatoid arthritis
- Trauma
- Muscle imbalances
- Poor body mechanics when exercising, such as during deep bench presses and dips
- Overtraining

Assessment

A doctor will conduct a health history and a physical evaluation asking you to perform a range of simple motions.

Treatment

- Rest
- NSAIDs
- Injections
- Home-based corrective physical therapy exercise (see page 52 for a frozen shoulder corrective exercise program)

ROTATOR CUFF INJURIES

The rotator cuff is made up of the subscapularis, infraspinatus, teres minor, and supraspinatus muscles, also known as the SITS muscles. The tendons of the four muscles merge to form the rotator cuff, which covers the top of the shoulder joint like a cuff and allows the shoulder to rotate in a full circle. An acute rotator cuff injury is very painful and occurs when a person falls on an outstretched arm. Chronic rotator cuff injuries usually occur due to gradual fraying of the tendons. If a rotator cuff injury is left unattended, it can worsen over time. Severe rotator cuff injuries may require surgery.

At the gym, people often focus only on the superficial, visible muscles while neglecting crucial, deep muscles like the SITS muscles that support and provide stabilization to the joint. The rotator cuff is responsible for internal and external rotation most commonly seen in throwing a ball or serving a tennis ball.

It was once thought that rotator cuff injuries were the result of sudden or severe trauma. It is now believed that degenerative changes occur over time as the result of misuse or abuse and may also be brought on by trauma.

Common Symptoms

- Pain during overhead motions such as reaching for something on a high shelf, combing your hair, and throwing a ball
- Pain when scratching your mid-back
- Pain when sleeping on your shoulder

Common Causes

Repetitive use and trauma are the most common mechanisms of a rotator cuff injury. Rotator cuff tears are seen quite often between the ages of 45 and 65. The most familiar repetitive injuries include poor execution of exercises in the weight room, lat pulls behind the neck or improper bench presses (see page 36 for common controversial exercises), and overuse with throwing sports. Rotator cuff injuries are also often the result of:

- Overuse tendinitis: Leads to irritation and fraying of the tendon
- Impingement tendinitis: The acromion can pinch and irritate the rotator cuff, or the bursa is swollen as a result of repetitive overhead motion.
- Calcification tendinitis: Inflammation can lead to calcium deposits within the rotator cuff.
- Severe tendinitis: Tears can cause partial or complete tearing of the rotator cuff.

Assessment

During your assessment, your doctor will take a health history, asking many questions about when your shoulder hurts and how you think you hurt it. Your doctor will perform a physical exam looking for signs of weakness, and he or she will listen for popping and grinding sounds. Often, the doctor will have you do the "soda can test," which is done by moving your arm as if pouring out soda. The doctor will gently resist the motion to determine the extent of the injury.

If a diagnosis cannot be made from the physical exam, the doctor may order imaging tests such as MRIs, x-rays, and arthrograms (dye is injected into the shoulder for this procedure).

Treatment

Generally, most doctors will try conservative care of rest, cold and heat packs, and medication. If that does not work, you may be referred to physical therapy, where corrective exercises along with ultrasound (gentle sound-wave vibrations) and electrical stimulation treatments may be administered. Some doctors will use cortisone injections to reduce the inflammation. If these fail to bring relief, surgical options may be discussed.

FROZEN SHOULDER

Frozen shoulder is called "adhesive capsulitis." A frozen shoulder can be the result of inflammation, scarring, thickening, or shrinkage of the joint capsule. This condition is often marked with stiffness or immobility due to the thickening of the shoulder capsule. When pain limits your movement, you'll generally reduce your range of motion. This allows adhesions to develop, and your shoulder "freezes." As these adhesions develop, they make movement even more difficult and painful—leading to further reduction of motion and a more frozen shoulder. This cycle of disuse sets up increased pain and immobility. Commonly reported injuries that lead to a frozen shoulder include tendinitis, bursitis, or a rotator cuff injury. Any long-term immobility of the shoulder region can lead to a frozen shoulder. Frozen shoulder conditions are more commonly seen in people between the ages of 40 and 70.

Common Symptoms

- Pain in all directions
- Reduced range of motion

Common Causes

- Insufficient movement
- Inflammation

- Adhesive capsulitis, where the shoulder capsule adheres to the head of the humerus

Assessment

During your assessment, your doctor will take a health history and conduct a physical exam.

Treatment

The objective is to increase motion and reduce pain. Your doctor may engage in aggressive joint mobilization along with stretching and electrical stimulation. They may also suggest the following options to treat your frozen shoulder:

- Gentle shoulder stretches
- Anti-inflammatory medications
- Mild and moist heat
- Ice applications
- Physical therapy or manual therapy and modalities
- Cortisone injections
- Surgical interventions

Also see the frozen shoulder corrective exercise program on page 52.

TENDINITIS AND BURSITIS

Tendinitis and bursitis are closely related and may occur alone or in combination. Tendinitis is inflammation of a tendon. In tendinitis of the shoulder, the rotator cuff and/or biceps tendon become inflamed, usually as a result of being pinched by surrounding structures. The injury may vary from mild inflammation to the swelling and thickening of most of the rotator cuff, which may then get trapped beneath the acromion. Tendinitis is often accompanied by inflammation of the bursa sacs that protect the shoulder. An inflamed bursa is called bursitis.

Common Symptoms

- The slow onset of discomfort and pain in the upper shoulder or upper third of the arm
- Difficulty sleeping on the shoulder
- Pain when the arm is forcefully pushed upward overhead

- Pain when the arm is lifted away from the body or overhead. If tendinitis involves the biceps tendon (the tendon located in front of the shoulder that helps bend the elbow and turn the forearm), pain will occur on the front or side of the shoulder and may travel down to the elbow and forearm.

Common Causes

- Repeated motion involving the arms
- Age
- Inflammation resulting from a disease such as rheumatoid arthritis
- Sports that overuse the shoulder
- Occupations requiring frequent overhead reaching

Assessment

Diagnosis of tendinitis and bursitis begins with a medical history and physical examination. X-rays do not show tendons or the bursa, but they may be helpful in ruling out bony abnormalities or arthritis. The doctor may remove and test fluid from the inflamed area to rule out infection.

Treatment

The majority of patients who see their doctor about a shoulder problem are there because of tendinitis. Most cases of tendinitis can be successfully treated. The first step is to reduce pain and inflammation with rest, ice, and anti-inflammatory medicines such as aspirin, naproxen, or ibuprofen. In some cases, the doctor or therapist will use ultrasound to warm deep tissues and improve blood flow. Before self-medicating, consult your doctor. Also, don't medicate yourself to cover up the pain so you can continue to play or work. While you may feel fine, you can be damaging the joint.

Gentle stretching and strengthening exercises are recommended and may be gradually added as you improve. The therapist may suggest applying a heat pack, engaging in gentle active motion, then applying an ice pack. If there is no improvement, the doctor may inject a corticosteroid medicine into the space under the acromion. While steroid injections are a common treatment, they must be used with caution because they can lead to tendon rupture. If there is still no improvement after 6 to 12 months, the doctor may perform either arthroscopic or open surgery to repair damage and relieve pressure on the tendons and bursae.

- Rest
- Heat and ice packs
- Medication

- Physical therapy
- Steroid injection

Also see the tendinitis and bursitis corrective exercise program on page 52.

THORACIC OUTLET SYNDROME (TOS)

Thoracic outlet syndrome, while not very common, is often misunderstood and misdiagnosed. The term first appeared in medical literature in 1956, in an article published by R. M. Peet and colleagues. It has been the subject of much controversy, and some experts say it is one of the most poorly understood, underdiagnosed, and misdiagnosed conditions.

TOS may be loosely defined as a group of disorders producing a constellation of signs and symptoms due to compression of blood vessels and nerves (neurovascular bundle) in the thoracic outlet region. The thoracic outlet is a space located between the rib cage (thorax) and the clavicle, which contains major blood vessels (subclavian artery and vein) and nerves (brachial plexus).

In general, the various groups of TOS (thoracic outlet syndrome) may be classified as follows:

True neurogenic TOS: Neurologic TOS is also called cervical rib and band syndrome. It usually affects one side of the body and predominantly occurs in women. Symptoms include weakness and atrophy of the hand, including the arm muscles, and intermittent aching, numbness, and paresthesia (burning or tingling sensation), which may also be felt in the fingers or arms. True neurogenic TOS may often be confused with carpal tunnel syndrome.

Traumatic TOS: As the name implies, this type of TOS occurs following trauma or injury. The most common type of trauma involves a fracture of the clavicle, which may also cause secondary injury to the nerves and blood vessels within the thoracic outlet. Traumatic TOS usually develops on the same side where the injury has occurred. The most frequent symptom is pain in the neck and shoulder area, which may be accompanied by weakness or numbness in the arm or hand.

Disputed TOS: This category of TOS is by far the most common type seen by doctors. The term "disputed TOS" (also known as nonspecific TOS) was applied to this disorder because its existence is controversial. The most prominent symptoms of disputed TOS include pain, paresthesia, and weakness. However, extensive clinical examination often fails to detect any objective evidence of an underlying problem or cause, which is why some experts have argued that this disorder does not exist. Proposed theories regarding the underlying cause of disputed TOS include trauma to the brachial plexus, congenital anomalies, or postural abnormalities.

True vascular TOS: This type of TOS involves damage to the subclavian artery or vein and can be documented by performing an arteriogram or venogram, which can reveal reduced blood flow to the area. Symptoms may include pain; numbness and coldness in the hands and fingers; and sores on the fingers. True vascular TOS is a rare disorder and may be caused by a congenital anomaly.

Common Symptoms

- Pain and a sense of numbness or tingling in the neck, shoulder, or arms
- Weakness, swelling, coldness, or a blue color in the arm or hand
- Neck or shoulder pain that may spread to the upper arm and forearm
- Weakness along the forearm, hand, and pinky
- Headaches stemming from the occipital or orbital areas
- Anterior chest wall pain (pseudo-angina)
- Wasting (atrophy) of the hand (in severe, chronic cases of TOS)

Common Causes

- Studies have shown that TOS is associated with jobs that incorporate heavy lifting and intense physical exertion (e.g., jackhammer operators, electricians, carpenters), as well as certain occupations that involve working in a static position for an extended period of time (e.g., secretaries, computer operators, bench workers). Both of these contribute to postural abnormalities.
- Trauma such as clavicle fractures, trauma to the shoulder, and hyperextension injuries of the neck (whiplash)
- Congenital anomaly (such as cervical rib and band syndrome, marked by the presence of abnormal fibromuscular bands present at birth that irritate or compress the brachial plexus)
- Postural distortions, such as drooping or sagging shoulders

Assessment

The following conditions, which produce signs and symptoms that may be confused with TOS, must be ruled out before a diagnosis of TOS can be considered:

- Carpal tunnel syndrome
- Cervical spine disease with nerve root compression
- Pancoast tumor (a type of lung tumor that grows in the thoracic inlet)
- Spinal cord tumor

- Degenerative spinal cord diseases (e.g., multiple sclerosis, syringomyelia)
- Other neuropathies (e.g., cubital tunnel syndrome, radial runnel compression)
- Tumor of the brachial plexus
- Inflammatory diseases of the shoulder (e.g., tendinitis, arthritis)
- Complex regional pain syndrome (e.g., reflex sympathetic dystrophy [RSD])
- Vascular diseases (e.g., atherosclerosis, thrombophlebitis)

A variety of diagnostic tests may be used in assessing patients with signs and symptoms of TOS. None of these tests are specific for TOS—they're used primarily to rule out other possible causes of symptoms that the patient experiences.

- Chest X-ray
- MRI of cervical spine
- CT scan of the brachial plexus
- Electromyography test used to measure muscle response to stimulation of nerves
- Nerve conduction studies
- Angiography of venography, if blood flow problems are suspected

Treatment

The objectives of treatment for patients with TOS include relieving and eliminating compression of the nerves and blood vessels in the thoracic outlet region; controlling and minimizing pain and other signs and symptoms associated with TOS; and improving the patient's overall quality of life. Most experts agree that a conservative approach is the first round of treatment in the management of patients with TOS unless the patient is experiencing significant neurologic impairment or acute vascular insufficiency due to neurovascular compression; in this case, surgery may be necessary. Approximately 85 percent of patients with TOS will improve with conservative treatment and only a small percentage of patients actually require surgery.

- Physical therapy (for corrective exercises, see the Specialized Corrective Exercise Programs on page 50).
- Muscle-strengthening exercises
- Stretching/isometric exercises
- Postural training to correct poor posture, such as drooping or sagging shoulders
- Osteopathic manipulation of the scalene and trapezius muscles

- Heat treatments with ultrasound

- Transcutaneous Electrical Nerve Stimulation (TENS) to control pain

- Swimming, although some authorities recommend avoiding the backstroke and breaststroke

- Drug therapy

- Analgesics and nonsteroidal anti-inflammatory drugs (NSAIDs) to reduce pain and inflammation

- Muscle relaxants to control muscle spasms

- Antidepressants (may be necessary for TOS patients with comorbid depression)

- Scalene injections with local anesthetic/steroid solutions to reduce pain

- Stellate ganglion block (may be given to patients with TOS who also have symptoms of RSD)

- Surgery

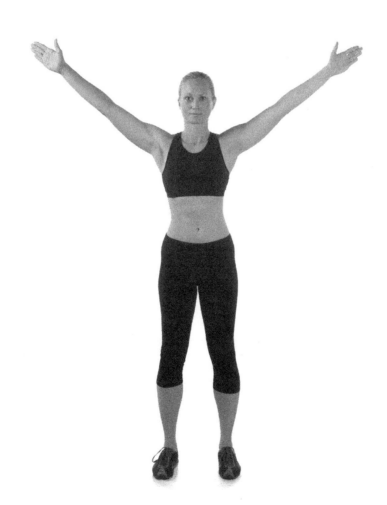

SHOULDER REHAB

You can greatly improve your chances of a full and rapid recovery by promptly visiting your doctor upon feeling pain, especially if you suffer from numbness in the hands and fingers or experience severe loss of function. Before starting any type of rehabilitation, have a doctor or therapist perform a complete evaluation of both your active range of motion (your ability to move your joint on your own) and passive range of motion (the ability of your health care provider to move your joint).

During the examination, the health care provider will compare the affected side to the unaffected side and evaluate the source, cause, and level of the shoulder pain as well as the range of motion and function. They will also perform a muscle test to ascertain which muscles are involved. The health care provider may order another exam, such as an MRI, before determining a course of therapy.

After a medical examination, you'll be given a diagnosis, which will indicate affected areas and the severity of injury. Knowing the cause of an injury is critical in developing a comprehensive rehabilitation program. Some injuries are the result of a sudden impact; others are the result of chronic

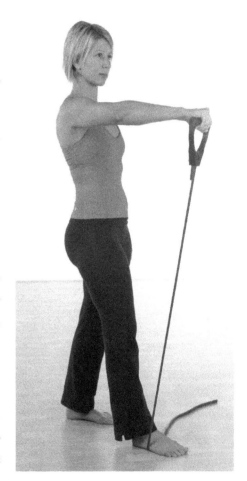

misuse, overuse, and abuse of the body or body parts. Generally speaking, there are two types of injury, macro trauma and micro trauma.

INJURY CLASSIFICATIONS

The three general classifications of injury are mild, moderate, and severe.

Mild. The doctor may recommend a home-based exercise program that includes corrective exercise and specific stretches. Keep in mind, you are still injured and reinjury is very common. Do not rush the body's healing.

Moderate. Passive and lightly active range-of-motion exercises may be advised to prevent a frozen shoulder. Protective rest of the joint, as well as modalities to control pain, will be recommended.

Severe. Rest, ice, and heat applications and range-of-motion exercises are often recommended. Pain-management options such as medication or injections can be discussed.

THE HEALING PROCESS

Once they make an accurate diagnosis, your therapist will design a treatment plan for your specific condition. The therapist will guide you along the steps, with your pain level and range of motion being key criteria for how much you should or shouldn't do.

Preventing further damage is critical. Attempting to "play through" pain and dismissing your injury will only prolong the rehabilitation process. Avoid movements such as overhead motions, sleeping on your affected side, or hanging your bag over your affected shoulder. Restoration of shoulder function should address both the local and general effects of the injury and comprehensively treat both the injury and the total person. Note that muscle strength can decrease up to 17 percent within the initial

72 hours of immobilization. The rate of decline slows after five to seven days, but muscle strength loss of up to 40 percent has been seen after six weeks of immobilization. The longer the immobilization period, the greater chance of soft tissue dysfunction and muscle atrophy, thus causing prolonged rehabilitation.

Note that the absence of symptoms does not mean full restoration. Just treating the injury and neglecting the total person will set you up for another injury. In athletes, 30 to 50 percent of all sports injuries are related to overuse or improper training techniques. Some studies have shown that 27 percent of these injuries are reinjuries, and that 16 percent occurred within one month of returning to play.

Also, remember the two-hour rule: If you hurt for more than two hours after an exercise session, you need to reduce activity to a level that does not cause pain; if you continue to hurt or lose range of motion, consult your doctor ASAP. An effective rehabilitation routine will train both the brain and the body, which is why you need to be mindful when training. In today's managed health care, physical therapists often don't have time to fully attend to all the aspects needed for complete restoration. This is why you play a significant part in restoring yourself to full function. Note: Do not mask your pain with medication. Pain is your body telling you that something is not right.

It's important to keep in mind that each person has his or her own timetable for recovery, and that the absence of pain is not a sign to return to "normal" activity. Also, many times people develop compensatory adjustments to make up for functional deficits, which may lead to further dysfunction further up or down the kinetic chain.

QUICK SHOULDER CARE TIPS

- Maintain proper posture.

- Motion is lotion—gently move your shoulder and arm several times each day.

- Avoid chills to the neck and shoulder area. Keep the joint area warm; warm joints are less easily injured and also respond better to movement than cold and stiff joints. Dressing in layers may be helpful.

- When sleeping on your side, rest the affected arm on top of a pillow for support.

- Avoid restrictive accessories that place pressure on the shoulder area (e.g., backpacks or heavy purses).

The rehabilitation goals occur in three stages: acute, recovery, and function.

PHASE 1: ACUTE STAGE

The acute stage focuses on preventing further harm, decreasing the signs and symptoms of injury, and hastening the healing process. A trained therapist should oversee this phase of rehabilitation.

The goals of Phase 1 are to:

- Manage pain
- Maintain range of motion
- Maintain neuromuscular control
- Prevent muscle atrophy

The criteria for advancement to Phase 2 are:

- Pain control
- Healing tissue
- Near-normal range of motion
- Tolerance for strength training

PHASE 2: RECOVERY PHASE

Follow the protocols set forth by a medical professional. At this stage, many people reinjure themselves, so be careful.

The goals of Phase 2 are to:

- Prevent further injury and pain
- Regain upper-body strength and muscular balance and stability
- Foster shoulder flexibility
- Improve neuromuscular control and coordination
- Evaluation for progression to next level

The criteria for advancement to Phase 3 are:

- No pain
- Complete tissue healing
- Almost complete range of motion
- Near-normal strength when compared to the uninvolved side (approximately 75 to 80 percent)

PHASE 3: FUNCTION PHASE

This phase can be done with an adaptive fitness personal trainer or on your own—as long as you follow the protocols set forth by a medical professional. Once you've regained full functional recovery, evaluate the circumstances that may have caused your condition and adapt your lifestyle and behaviors. By being sensible, following your therapist's suggestions, and participating in the exercises included in this book, you reduce your chances of reinjuring yourself.

The goals of Phase 3 are to:

- Learn the importance of proper training techniques
- Learn how to exercise the stabilizing muscles
- Learn proper posture and lifestyle changes to prevent future injury
- Increase muscular strength and endurance in preparation for work or sports demands
- Improve multiplane range of motion
- Institute sport-specific drills and functional activities of daily living
- Evaluation prior to reengage in a fully active lifestyle

The criteria for knowing you've reached full functional recovery are:

- Zero pain
- Full and complete pain-free range of motion and flexibility
- Strength equal to the uninvolved side
- Normal body mechanics

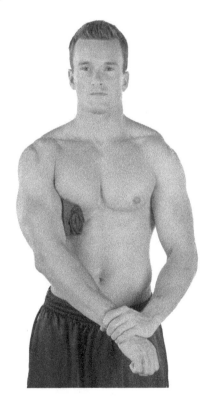

PART 2

PREVENTIVE AND SPECIALIZED PROGRAMS

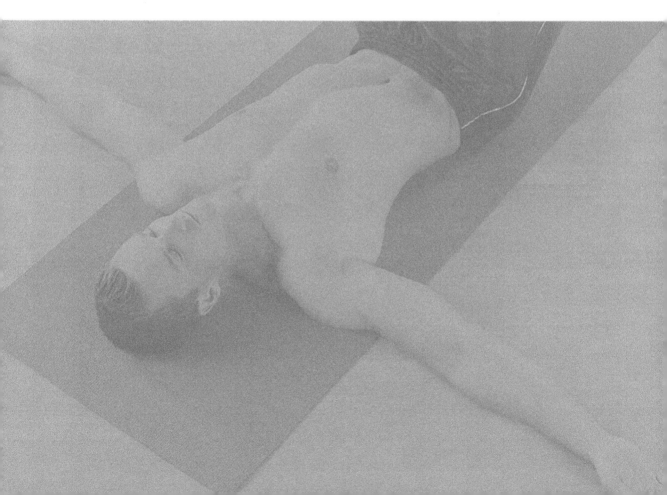

PREVENTING (RE)INJURY

We're all familiar with the saying "An ounce of prevention is worth a pound of cure." We all understand that preventing a problem is a wise idea. This concept is just as relevant in protecting our shoulder joint as it is in maintaining our automobile, whether it's with a regular oil change or tune-up. Preventive maintenance can ward off a breakdown or an expensive repair. Unfortunately, when it comes to our bodies, we oftentimes neglect that basic idea.

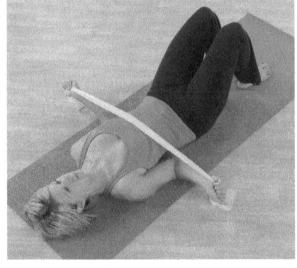

Let's assume you've recovered from a shoulder injury or are on your way to full function. Staying proactive provides the best defense against a recurring shoulder problem. Ask your doctor how to best use heat and ice. Most therapists suggest moist heat to loosen a joint, followed by active warm-up to foster improved range of motion, followed by ice after activity. It is common to apply cold in the case of an acute injury.

You should also begin a comprehensive shoulder-conditioning program with a specific stretching routine. While strength training is a good thing, too much can cause excessive tightness and possible injury. While stretching is good, too much can lead to a lax joint and possible reinjury. Remember: More is not always better! Joseph Pilates (the father of Pilates exercises) said it best: "Stretch what is tight, strengthen what is lax."

The exercises in Part 3 of this book have been selected from a review of the best therapeutic exercise publications addressing the shoulder. Treat this book as a menu from which you (either in consultation with your health care professional or simple experimentation) select appropriate exercises for your condition. If you've had physical therapy, you might even recognize some of these exercises. You can approach the exercises in a proactive manner, but if you notice that you're manifesting some shoulder concerns, it's always wise to talk to your health care provider. Otherwise, start with the gentlest exercise and progress from there.

Here are some basic guidelines to follow when determining which exercises to do. If in doubt, consult with your health care provider.

If you've had chronic or recurrent shoulder instabilities, ask your health care provider if you can do:

- Isometric exercises to increase internal and external muscles
- Resistance tube exercises

(You may need to wear a protective device to limit your shoulder motions.)

If you've experienced shoulder impingement, you should:

- Relearn proper body mechanics.
- Strengthen rotator cuff muscles.
- Strengthen lower extremities to reduce shoulder strain when throwing.
- Be alert to what caused the incident and be careful. If you're over 40, be especially mindful. Use RICE—rest, ice, compression, elevation—when needed.

If you've had bursitis, you should:

- Avoid overuse.
- Maintain flexibility.

If you have arthritis, you should:

- Avoid overuse.
- Balance strengthening exercises with flexibility exercises.

You'll also find sample programs for common activities starting on page 43.

POSTURE'S ROLE IN PREVENTION

Most people know that poor posture can lead to back pain, but posture also plays an important role in shoulder health. For instance, the rounded-shoulder, forward-head posture (think turtle) is often seen in people who swim a lot using the crawl/freestyle stroke without strengthening the opposing muscle group and stretching the chest muscles. This decreased flexibility of the chest and shoulder can set the stage for shoulder problems. Experts now understand that if one body part is misaligned, overused, or hurt, it can affect the mechanics somewhere along the kinetic chain.

Look for the image of good posture below. Notice that her ear, shoulder, hip, and ankle are all on the same vertical line. Any deviation from this alignment can lead to a multitude of issues, from neck and shoulder problems to lower-back pain. Of course, plenty of things, like working a desk job, sitting in a cramped airplane seat, and fixing a car, will challenge your ability to maintain good posture. That's why you should assess your posture several times a day.

The easiest way to do this is to stand with your back against a wall, with your heels no more than 6 inches from the wall. Place your bottom to the wall then attempt to place your upper back and the base of your head to the wall, keeping your chin down. If you have very compromised posture, start with just placing your bottom against the wall; as you improve, take your time trying to get your upper back against the wall before finally attempting to get your head to the wall. Some older people with severely compromised posture never get their head to the wall, so start today before it's too late. Practicing proper posture will reduce issues in all parts of the body, from head to toe.

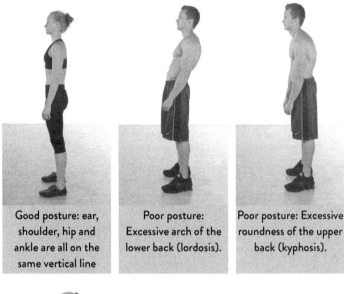

Good posture: ear, shoulder, hip and ankle are all on the same vertical line

Poor posture: Excessive arch of the lower back (lordosis).

Poor posture: Excessive roundness of the upper back (kyphosis).

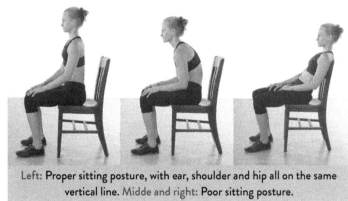

Left: Proper sitting posture, with ear, shoulder and hip all on the same vertical line. Midde and right: Poor sitting posture.

THE GREEN, YELLOW, AND RED ZONES

Too often people hurt their shoulder because they're not paying attention to how they're using it. If you've had a shoulder injury before, you should be particularly careful. One movement that commonly triggers a shoulder problem is simply reaching too far behind your "safe" zone. By staying mindful of the green, yellow, and red zone concept, you can prevent further shoulder issues. The zones relate to three kinds of shoulder/arm movements: opening your arms (abduction), lifting your arms forward (flexion), and taking your arms backward (extension). Note that each arm/shoulder may have a different comfort zone and that changing hand position (e.g., turning your palms up, facing them inward) can affect mobility in one or both shoulders.

Most people can perform movements in the green zone. The green zone places the least amount of stress on your shoulder and should be sufficient when doing any activity, including exercise and rehabilitation. When your elbow/hand is in the yellow zone, there is moderate stress on your shoulder; caution should be used in this zone. When you reach into the red zone, the shoulder is under the most stress, making it unstable and vulnerable to injury. Try to avoid motions in the red zone when possible, especially if you have an injured shoulder.

To determine your zones when abducting your arms, start by standing with your back against a wall.

1. Raise your arms in front of you at shoulder height with your palms facing each other. Now spread them to just where you can't see your hands anymore. Does this hurt? If not, this is your green zone—you can perform most activities in this zone and not hurt yourself.

2. Now spread your hands back to the wall. Does this hurt? This is the yellow zone— this is where some people display tightness. Whether or not you feel tightness, you should still be careful in this zone.

3. The red zone is behind you, such as when you reach into the back seat of the car without turning your body.

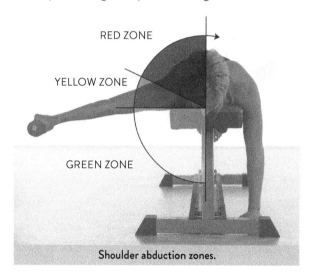

RED ZONE

YELLOW ZONE

GREEN ZONE

Shoulder abduction zones.

To determine your zones when moving your arms forward (shoulder flexion), start by standing with your arms alongside your body.

1. Raise your arms forward to shoulder height with your palms facing each other. This area should move freely and is your green zone.

2. As you raise your arms above shoulder height, you may feel some restriction. This is your yellow zone.

3. Anything above and beyond your head is the red zone.

To determine your zones when moving your arms backward (shoulder extension), start by standing with your arms alongside your body.

1. Slowly move your arms straight back 3–4 inches. This should feel relatively comfortable and is your green zone.

2. The difference between the yellow and red zones is very small, so be careful any time you move your arm back and up (to scratch your upper back, for instance).

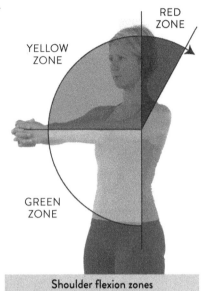

Shoulder flexion zones

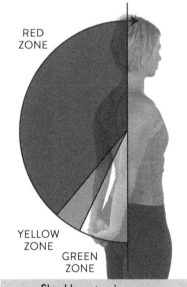

Shoulder extension zones

Following these Do's and Don'ts can dramatically reduce shoulder injury:

Do's

- Separate and lighten loads.

- Lift and carry loads close to your body.

- Take frequent breaks from any repetitious activity.

- Sleep on your back or your unaffected shoulder with a pillow between your arm and body. Watch that your shoulder stays in line with your body. You might also rest your affected arm on top of a pillow.

- Wear a fanny pack, sling your bag's strap across your body and unaffected shoulder, or tuck the load between your body and elbow.

- When performing activities that are shoulder intensive, such as sweeping or vacuuming, move your whole body by moving your feet and keep your arm tucked in close to your side. Take small steps and keep your back straight.

- Use inexpensive grabber devices to protect your shoulder.

- Practice good posture.

- Rearrange your workstation.

- Alternate the arm you use to carry your briefcase or purse.

- Pay close attention to how your head and upper back are positioned while at work and during activities of daily living.

- Make sure you're not placing too much load in your arms when you're sitting at your desk or workstation.

Don'ts

- Don't slump and let your shoulder round forward.

- Don't work with your arms overhead for prolonged periods.

- Don't lift excessively heavy loads.

- Don't allow your hands to be out of your sight when your arms are out to the side.

- Don't reach far in front or in back of you to pick something up.

- Don't work for more than 15–20 minutes without a rest break for your shoulder.

- Don't sleep on your affected shoulder.

- Don't sling the strap of your purse or other load over your affected shoulder.

- Don't prop yourself up on your affected arm while reading or watching TV.

- Don't rest your affected arm on the car-door window ledge.

- Don't carry heavy bags or purses on your shoulders.

- Don't overdo it in activities in which you normally don't participate. Train to play.

CONTROVERSIAL EXERCISES

Everyone knows that physical activity and exercise is good for the human body. Unfortunately, in our zest to get fit, we often hurt ourselves because we're using outdated principles or are driven by faulty assumptions. The fitness industry has evolved, but some exercises have been around so long that it seems irreverent to question their efficacy.

Many of us are bombarded with glitzy infomercials and celebrity endorsements that convey erroneous exercise facts. Successful coaches who have produced winning teams have also passed down some faulty myths. Often, training methods get adopted and later institutionalized based on anecdotal information rather than science.

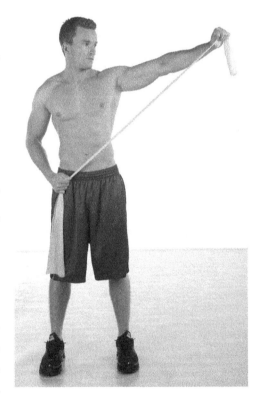

Most of the controversial exercises discussed here will not kill you today or even really hurt you if done once or twice. The problem is cumulative and manifests itself over time. The human body is resilient, but if it's constantly misused and abused, the negative effects of improper exercise will show up in later years.

One expert stated that at least 90 percent of exercise programs include some exercises that are as detrimental as they are valuable. The key when determining if an exercise is correct is whether or not it passes the benefits-to-risk ratio: Ask yourself if this exercise is doing more harm than good, and is there a safer, more effective way to get the desired results? You should also be mindful when selecting an activity/sport or a piece of equipment.

Before embarking on an activity, ask yourself the following:

- Why am I doing this exercise/activity?
- What are the benefits vs. risk of this exercise/activity?
- How do I feel while doing this exercise/activity?
- How do I feel after doing this exercise/activity?
- Could I receive the same benefits doing a different exercise/activity?
- Is the activity biomechanically correct?
- Does it accomplish what I want it to?
- Does the exercise work the targeted muscle?
- Is it harming a joint?
- Train, don't strain!

SHOULDER JOINT CONSIDERATIONS

Areas prone to injury are the shoulders, knees, lower back, and neck. Stay alert to the variables discussed here and you'll avoid a cervical neck, upper-back, or shoulder problem.

According to orthopedic doctors, shoulder impingement is increasingly becoming a concern for exercisers. All movements involving the shoulder region need to be controlled, and the hands should be supinated (palms up) if raising the arms above shoulder height as this allows more space in the joint. Using hand weights with the arms fully extended can aggravate shoulder problems and may cause elbow problems as well. Relax the shoulders and retract the shoulder blades when performing arm exercises (there is a tendency to shrug the shoulders up near the ears when exercising the arms).

You know how your body feels—listen to it and heed what it says.

Do not become complacent about exercise, especially if you've suffered an injury. It's critical for you to be mindful of proper body mechanics when working out and to associate with your body while working out. This involves paying attention to what you're doing and how the exercise affects your body. One thought to consider is not playing music while exercising because it's easy to forget about your form. Once the move is in your muscle memory, you can use music, but still focus on form. Remember: Only perfect practice makes perfect! Think PP, which stands for Perfect Posture. The key to injury prevention is to exercise smart, not hard. Any exercise that has made it into your routine should give maximum return on your investment.

Any exercise done incorrectly can cause problems, but some common exercises are riskier than others. The following 13 exercises fail the "benefits to risk" index:

1. Lat pulls when the bar is pulled down behind the neck or done too quickly and pulled down far below chin level.

2. Military presses done behind the head/neck.

3. Dumbbell flys and reverse flys done with the arms extremely wide (i.e., in the yellow and red zones).

4. Bench presses with barbell or dumbbells held too wide or with the elbows dipping too far below or behind the bench. Placing the hands in a more neutral grip puts less strain on the shoulder.

5. Lateral raises and frontal raises done too quickly or lifted higher than shoulder height.

6. Upright rows when the bar is pulled too high.

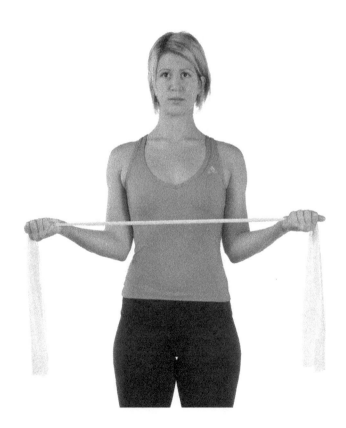

7. Shrugs when done with improper grip width (too wide or too narrow) or when shoulders roll forward and drop quickly. Shrugs when performed with a comfortable weight are okay.

8. Bicep curls done on a straight barbell. Instead, use a neutral grip. Dumbbells would be a better choice when doing bicep curls.

9. Triceps curls done with machines or performed with awkward positioning (e.g., French curls).

10. Wide-grip pull-ups and pull-ups done behind the head.

11. The use of water exercise equipment or movements that replicate contraindicated weight exercises. While water exercise is generally excellent and low impact, poor biomechanics and classes taught by ill-trained instructors can hurt you. In the water, the 3 S's determine resistance: size of the object, speed of the movement, and shape of the object.

12. Push-ups when done too wide or done in a manner that strains your shoulder. Push-ups done with hands in a neutral position are best.

13. Bar dips done too low or too quickly.

BE CAREFUL

High-risk areas besides the shoulder include the knees, neck, lower back, hips, and ankles. Pay special attention to these areas when implementing exercises.

Stay alert to the variables discussed here and you'll avoid a cervical neck, upper-back, or shoulder problem.

DESIGNING A SHOULDER ROUTINE

If you've read this book from the beginning, you'll have learned all about the shoulder's amazing mobility as well as its areas of vulnerability. The range of activities that could negatively affect the shoulder might even be discouraging to you.

However, rather than giving up on swimming, playing tennis, or even painting your kitchen, you can continue doing what you enjoy by conditioning your body and maintaining a high level of fitness. Giving your shoulder a simple daily dose of TLC will provide a big return on investment.

Part 3 features a number of exercises designed to help you recover from an injury or maintain a healthy shoulder. Every effort was made to include only movements and exercises recognized by shoulder experts and therapists. If you're in the early stages of your rehabilitation, you should follow your medical professional's recommendations to the letter for the best results. The exercises they prescribe may or may not be in this book, and that's fine. If you've fully recovered

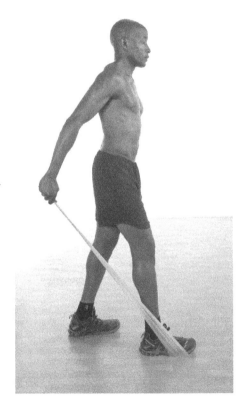

and have been discharged by your doctor, go ahead and select the exercises that appeal to you, changing them up periodically.

The advantage of having this book is that you can take it with you to your therapist and ask her/him to highlight the exercises they'd like you to do and the ones you should avoid. It's important to remember that there is no perfect exercise for everyone, nor is there a perfect training routine. In functional fitness, everything should be adapted and individualized for your specific needs. This book can be a living document that will allow you to monitor, add, and delete exercises as are appropriate.

The exercises you choose should be specific, purposeful, and goal oriented, with each movement contained within the program leading to greater independence and normalized function. Functional shoulder exercises should follow this progression:

- Large muscles to small muscles
- Simple movements to complex motions
- Static movements to dynamic motions
- Slow movements to fast motions
- Movements in a single plane to movements in multiple planes
- Low-force activities to high-force activities
- Dual-arm movements to single-arm motions
- Stable-surface drills to stability challengers

If you're in recovery mode, trial and error is the best approach. Start slowly and include some basic active exercises and stretches as well as a few corrective exercises. If you notice an increase in your symptoms, stop immediately and consult your health advisor.

If you don't have an existing shoulder issue, follow this basic protocol:

Stretches

- Beginners: Hold each stretch for 10–15 seconds.
- Advanced: Hold each stretch for up to 1 minute.

Active Exercises

- Beginners: Start with 5 repetitions (reps).
- Advanced: Work up to 15 reps, then move on to another pain-free exercise.

As always, remember to warm up first and aim for quality motions over quantity. Before advancing to the next level, you should be able to correctly perform the skill's previous level. Advancing too quickly just because you're bored increases your risks for a possible reinjury. Therapeutic exercises are not about increasing the load or length of stretch time each time—in this case, more is not better.

Whether or not you're nursing an existing injury, if you experience any increase in pain or symptoms, such as numbness or tingling, do not continue with any exercise from this book and consult your doctor. Your doctor's advice supersedes the information in this book because of his or her familiarity with your unique situation.

EXERCISE SAFETY TIPS

Early intervention to identify a problem keeps small problems small.

- Maintain a proper balance between training and proper rest.

- Balance your volume of training with intensity of training.

- Know your range of motion. Each of us has a unique range of motion of the shoulder—learn your safe range. One person's range may be another person's pain.

- Learn which exercises are high-risk exercises as they pertain to your shoulder.

- Always perform your exercises with proper execution.

- Learn various methods to cross-train to prevent overuse syndrome. Don't overtrain the same muscles in the same manner day in and day out (e.g., swimming for yards and yards every day).

- Always include exercises to train the small supporting muscles of your shoulder. Most of us focus on the "show" muscles and forget the importance of these smaller muscles.

- Understand the possible dangers of too many speed movements in your activity.

- Train smart, NOT heavy. Too much weight combined with poor execution equals injury!

- Understand how to mix reps and sets for maximum gain and minimum risk.

- Learn how to prepare for activity, whether it's preseason conditioning or pregame joint readiness.

SAMPLE CONDITIONING PROGRAMS

This section features shoulder programs for several sports, occupations, and common shoulder conditions. It also includes a program for general overall conditioning. Assuming you are pain free, locate the program that applies to you and perform it daily; a cross-training approach in which you stretch daily and do the conditioning exercises 2–3 times a week might also work well. Prior to doing any exercise, remember to warm up the joint area. A warm-up is not the same as stretching—a warm-up is simply any activity that increases muscle temperature so the joint is more limber. Tight muscles, ligaments, and tendons are more inclined to be injured.

Determining how long to hold a stretch or how many reps to do is truly an individual decision. There is no magic formula that will work for everyone. Each person will respond differently, and remember the old adage "let pain be your guide" has never been more applicable than with shoulder treatment. Avoid overdoing it; more is not always better. The bottom line is your shoulder will tell you how high to reach, how far to stretch, and how long to hold a stretch.

However, if you don't have an existing shoulder issue, you can follow the basic protocol noted on page 44. Some of the programs will suggest strengthening exercises that utilize a band or dumbbell. If you have one but not the other, feel free to do the exercise with the prop you have on hand.

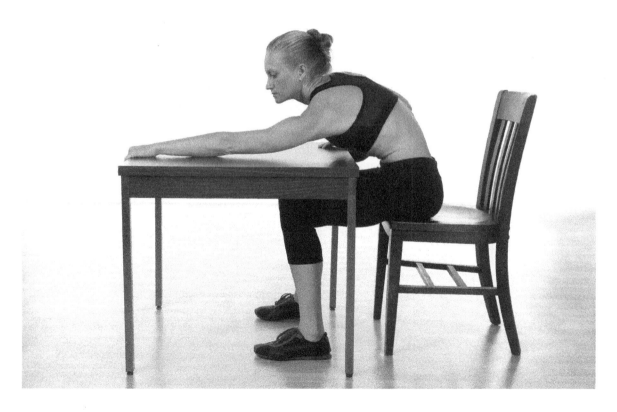

GENERAL CONDITIONING

This program is designed to provide overall wellness to the shoulder complex. You won't build giant muscles or extreme flexibility doing these exercises; you'll simply keep your shoulders in good working order and prevent injuries from occurring. This program can be easily integrated into your usual exercise routine.

These exercises should be done after a thermal warm-up or after your workout.

STRETCH

Choker, *p. 65*

Arm Pulls, *p. 68*

Corner Stretch, *p. 109*

Shoulder Blade Pinch, *p. 74*

Beginners: Hold 10–15 seconds.
Advanced: Hold up to 1 minute.

ACTIVE EXERCISE

Shoulder Rolls, *p. 59*

Elbow Touches, *p. 60*

Serving Tray, *p. 131*

Internal Rotation with Band, *p. 132*

Beginners: Start with 5 reps.
Advanced: Work up to 15 reps.

BASEBALL/SOFTBALL

Rotator cuff injuries and shoulder impingement concerns are the most common shoulder problems seen in throwing sports. Baseball pitchers have a higher incidence of shoulder problems than softball pitchers due to the mechanics of the pitch. However, infielders who do a great deal of repetitive infield work are at risk in both sports. To prevent an injury, begin conditioning well before the preseason period to prepare your body for hours of throwing.

STRETCH

Choker, *p. 65*

Over the Top, *p. 66*

Chest Stretch (Doorway), *p. 110*

Beginners: Hold 10–15 seconds.
Advanced: Hold up to 1 minute.

ACTIVE EXERCISE

Pendulum (Forward and Backward), *p. 55*

T's with Band, *p. 139*

Internal Rotation with Band, *p. 132*

External Rotation with Band, *p. 133*

Dumbbell Shoulder Extension, *p. 142*

Dumbbell Soup Can Pours, *p. 143*

Beginners: Start with 5 reps.
Advanced: Work up to 15 reps.

BASKETBALL

Although lower-body injuries are more common in basketball players, shoulder issues can still pop up when players aren't paying attention. Shooting too many baskets over a short period of time, such as early in the preseason, may result in rotator cuff tendinitis. Falls that can lead to injury are also common in basketball.

STRETCH

Choker, *p. 65*

Over the Top, *p. 66*

Chest Stretch (Doorway), *p. 110*

> **Beginners:** Hold 10–15 seconds.
> **Advanced:** Hold up to 1 minute.

ACTIVE EXERCISE

Pendulum (Forward and Backward), *p. 55*

T's with Band, *p. 139*

Internal Rotation with Band, *p. 132*

External Rotation with Band, *p. 133*

Dumbbell Shoulder Extension, *p. 142*

Dumbbell Soup Can Pours, *p. 143*

> **Beginners:** Start with 5 reps.
> **Advanced:** Work up to 15 reps.

FOOTBALL

Shoulder dislocations are common in football. Preseason conditioning should consist of strengthening the shoulder complex to provide as much stability and support as possible to the shoulder girdle and joint area. This, plus a dose of good luck, is critical to stay injury free.

STRETCH

Choker, *p. 65*

Over the Top, *p. 66*

Chest Stretch (Doorway), *p. 110*

> **Beginners:** Hold 10–15 seconds.
> **Advanced:** Hold up to 1 minute.

ACTIVE EXERCISE

Pendulum (Forward and Backward), *p. 55*

Dumbbell Reverse Fly, *p. 144*

Internal Rotation with Band, *p. 132*

External Rotation with Band, *p. 133*

> **Beginners:** Start with 5 reps.
> **Advanced:** Work up to 15 reps.

GOLF

Golf might look like a gentle enough sport, but when played often or without proper technique, it can lead to injury from overuse or misuse. While shoulder issues appear less frequently in golfers than back, elbow, hand, and wrist problems, some experience rotator cuff impingement.

The following should be done prior to playing golf and in between holes.

STRETCH

Reverse Lift, *p. 96*

Picture Frame, *p. 63*

Upper-Back Stretch, *p. 72*

Beginners: Hold 10–15 seconds
Advanced: Hold up to 1 minute.

ACTIVE EXERCISE

Pendulum (Across Body), *p. 56*

Shoulder Box, *p. 58*

Elbow Touches (Supine), *p. 82*

Straight-Arm Stretch, *p. 84*

Shoulder Slaps, *p. 102*

I's, Y's, and T's on Roller, *p. 103*

Beginners: Start with 5 reps.
Advanced: Work up to 15 reps.

HOCKEY

The majority of hockey injuries result from direct trauma, whether through falls or player contact. Knee, hand, and wrist injuries are the most common, but players are also subject to shoulder separations/dislocations. The best prevention for this is to strengthen the shoulder muscles as well as maintain flexibility.

STRETCH

Choker, *p. 65*

Over the Top, *p. 66*

Chest Stretch (Doorway), *p. 110*

Beginners: Hold 10–15 seconds.
Advanced: Hold up to 1 minute.

ACTIVE EXERCISE

Shoulder Box, *p. 58*

Elbow Touches, *p. 60*

Dumbbell Reverse Fly, *p. 144*

Beginners: Start with 5 reps.
Advanced: Work up to 15 reps.

SWIMMING

Any sport that requires repetitive overhead motions has a high risk of injury. In swimming, the freestyle/crawl, backstroke, and butterfly present the most risk. Strokes done with an underwater recovery, such as the breaststroke, are easier on the shoulder.

Consider doing underwater recovery strokes during rehab, and focus on techniques, kicks, and quality workouts rather than high-volume workouts.

STRETCH

Choker, *p. 65*

Over the Top, *p. 66*

Chest Stretch (Doorway), *p. 110*

Internal Rotation Stretch, *p. 67*

The Zipper, *p. 80*

Beginners: Hold 10–15 seconds.
Advanced: Hold up to 1 minute.

ACTIVE EXERCISE

Shoulder Box, *p. 58*

Elbow Touches, *p. 60*

Shoulder Extension, *p. 125*

External Rotation with Band, *p. 133*

Beginners: Start with 5 reps.
Advanced: Work up to 15 reps.

TENNIS

Tennis requires flexibility and power. Tennis serves count on the shoulder joint to perform at high speeds and at extreme ranges of motion. This combination sets the stage for bursitis and rotator cuff injuries. The backhand can also place the shoulder joint in awkward angles.

STRETCH

Choker, *p. 65*

Over the Top, *p. 66*

The Zipper, *p. 80*

Beginners: Hold 10–15 seconds.
Advanced: Hold up to 1 minute.

ACTIVE EXERCISE

Pendulum (Across Body), *p. 56*

Soup Can Pours, *p. 71*

Serving Tray, *p. 131*

Shoulder Extension, *p. 125*

Sword Fighter, *p. 128*

External Rotation with Band, *p. 133*

Beginners: Start with 5 reps.
Advanced: Work up to 15 reps.

VOLLEYBALL

Volleyball players who serve and spike are at greater risk of injury than those who set the ball. Also, due to the nature of the sport, players are constantly diving for the ball on the beach or the gym floor. This presents opportunities for shoulder dislocation.

STRETCH

Choker, *p. 65*

Over the Top, *p. 66*

Beginners: Hold 10–15 seconds.
Advanced: Hold up to 1 minute.

ACTIVE EXERCISE

T's with Band, *p. 139*

Y's with Band, *p. 138*

Sword Fighter, *p. 128*

Prone Crossing Guard, *p. 148*

Dumbbell Soup Can Pours, *p. 143*

Beginners: Start with 5 reps.
Advanced: Work up to 15 reps.

WRESTLING OR MIXED MARTIAL ARTS

Wrestling exposes players to major impact that can result in dislocations. Additionally, wrestlers' arms are commonly placed or forced in unnatural positions that overstretch the shoulder joint. Wrestlers need adequate strength and power along with flexibility in order to not get injured when they're stretched and pulled like Gumby.

STRETCH

Choker, *p. 65*

Over the Top, *p. 66*

Chest Stretch (Doorway), *p. 110*

Beginners: Hold 10–15 seconds.
Advanced: Hold up to 1 minute.

ACTIVE EXERCISE

Shoulder Box, *p. 58*

Elbow Touches, *p. 60*

Dumbbell Reverse Fly, *p. 144*

Beginners: Start with 5 reps.
Advanced: Work up to 15 reps.

CONSTRUCTION JOB

In construction, a worker's body is oftentimes also his tool. Workers who perform a lot of overhead work are at an increased risk for shoulder problems so they should take special care to do these exercises when they're not on the job.

STRETCH

Choker, *p. 65*

Over the Top, *p. 66*

Chest Stretch (Doorway), *p. 110*

Internal Rotation Stretch, *p. 67*

The Zipper, *p. 80*

Beginners: Hold 10–15 seconds.
Advanced: Hold up to 1 minute.

ACTIVE EXERCISE

Shoulder Box, *p. 58*

Elbow Touches, *p. 60*

Dumbbell Shoulder Extension, *p. 142*

External Rotation with Band, *p. 133*

Beginners: Start with 5 reps.
Advanced: Work up to 15 reps.

OFFICE/DESK JOB

While sitting at a desk all day isn't particularly strenuous, it can place your body in awkward positions for long periods of time. Pay attention to whether or not you hunch over paperwork or move around a mouse at an ergonomically incorrect workstation. Shoulder pain may accompany common desk-job ailments such as neck strain and carpal tunnel syndrome, so remember to get up and stretch a few times an hour and be vigilant about keeping good posture.

STRETCH

Choker, *p. 65*

Over the Top, *p. 66*

Chest Stretch (Doorway), *p. 110*

Beginners: Hold 10–15 seconds.
Advanced: Hold up to 1 minute.

CORRECTIVE EXERCISE

Pendulum (Forward and Backward), *p. 55*

T's with Band, *p. 139*

Internal Rotation with Band, *p. 132*

External Rotation with Band, *p. 133*

Dumbbell Shoulder Extension, *p. 142*

Dumbbell Soup Can Pours, *p. 143*

Beginners: Start with 5 reps.
Advanced: Work up to 15 reps.

SPECIALIZED CORRECTIVE EXERCISE PROGRAMS

This section includes corrective exercises for all of the shoulder conditions listed earlier in the text.

Studies have shown that for people with persistent shoulder pain, exercise therapy is an excellent adjunct to injections or surgery, long term. In addition to shoulder exercises, manual therapy can help decrease pain and improve shoulder mobility.

After an injury or surgery, a corrective exercise conditioning program may help you return to your activities of daily living and enjoy life more fully. A corrective shoulder conditioning program should provide a wide range of exercises. The goal is functional fitness, or trying to match the movements to your daily functions. This term is often used in therapy.

Before embarking on any exercise program, consult your health care provider to match the exercises to your condition. Remember more is not always better–train smart! A comprehensive corrective exercise program for the shoulder should address strengthening the shoulder joint and a safe flexibility routine that restores range of motion.

Experts in the field of shoulder rehabilitation suggest that a comprehensive program include the prime movers and supporting muscles, such as: deltoids; trapezius; rhomboid; teres major and minor; supraspinatus and infraspinatus; and subscapularis.

SHOULDER IMPINGEMENT

Internal Rotation (Supine), *p. 89*

Rotator Cuff (External Rotation), *p. 81*

Shrug, *p. 141*

Elbow Touches, *p. 60*

Choker, *p. 65*

Shoulder Box, *p. 58*

Picture Frame, *p. 63*

Another option for people who have arthritis of the shoulder is water exercise. Water exercise allows for the advantage of gentle movements throughout the full range of motion. For more detained corrective exercises within the pool, check out *Make the Pool Your Gym*, published by Ulysses Press.

REPETITIVE INJURY SERIES

Chest Stretch (Doorway), *p. 110*

Choker, *p. 65*

Over the Top, *p. 66*

Internal Rotation Stretch, *p. 67*

The Zipper, *p. 80*

ROTATOR CUFF INJURIES

Downward Sword Fighter, *p. 127*

External Rotation with Band, *p. 133*

Rotator Cuff (External Rotation), *p. 81*

External Rotation (Wall), *p. 115*

Internal Rotation with Band, *p. 132*

Pull-Downs, *p. 135*

Seated Rowing, *p. 134*

Sword Fighter, *p. 128*

Shrug, *p. 141*

Over the Top, *p. 66*

Shoulder Rolls, *p. 59*

Picture Frame, *p. 63*

TENDINITIS AND BURSITIS

Dumbbell Reverse Fly, *p. 144*

Sword Fighter, *p. 128*

Downward Sword Fighter, *p. 127*

Seated Rowing, *p. 134*

Pull-Downs, *p. 135*

Elbow Touches, *p. 60*

Shoulder Box, *p. 58*

Choker, *p. 65*

Serving Tray, *p. 131*

SHOULDER DISLOCATIONS

Pendulum (Forward and Backward), *p. 55*

Internal Rotation with Band, *p. 132*

External Rotation with Band, *p. 133*

Beginners: Start with 5 reps.
Advanced: Work up to 15 reps.

FROZEN SHOULDER

Arm Swing Series, *p. 55–57*

Pendulum (Forward and Backward), *p. 55*

Hanging Arm Circles, *p. 57*

Finger Walking (Forward), *p. 105*

Finger Walking (Side), *p. 106*

Internal Rotation option with or without Band, *p. 132*

External Rotation option with or without Band, *p. 133*

Sword Fighter, *p. 128*

Serving Tray, *p. 131*

Always perform a shoulder warm-up before embarking on an exercise program. Good options are a warm shower or bath for a few minutes, or applying a moist heating pad.

PART 3

SHOULDER CONDITIONING EXERCISES

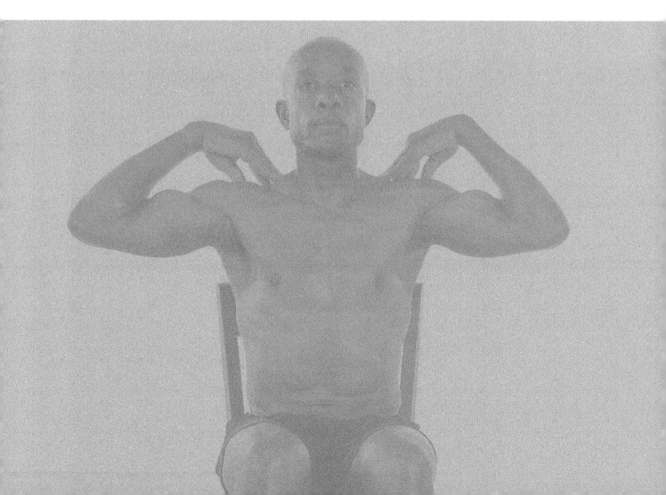

THE EXERCISES

The exercises in this chapter are grouped according to the position in which the exercise is performed, or its purpose. For instance, exercises that are done while standing are presented together. Generally, the exercises are listed in progression from easiest to most challenging. While the focus of each exercise is to restore function to your affected shoulder, it is advised that you perform the exercises bilaterally to prevent an injury to the other shoulder.

As you embark on the recovery process, you need to become your own personal trainer. The goal of a good trainer is to do NO harm. As a good trainer, you need to train smart—not hard. Avoid any activity that aggravates your shoulder. Pain is your body's way of informing you that something is going on internally. Never mask your pain with medications or lotions. To prevent a reinjury or unnecessary pain, execute motions with proper form.

THE TWO-HOUR RULE

If your body hurts more than two hours post-workout, you did too much and need to rest until you can find a workout that is pain free. If you suspect a reinjury, schedule a follow-up appointment with your doctor ASAP. Speak with your doctor/therapist about how and when you should heat and/or ice the affected area. "No pain, no gain" is insane! Listen to your body and heed what it says. Exercise only to tolerance level.

PASSIVE AND GENTLE SERIES

Prior to performing these motions, externally warm up the shoulder area, either by taking a warm shower or applying a moist heat pack. Consult your doctor first as to how you should warm up the joint. Use caution when applying heat to the area to avoid a burn. Please note: Generally a safe place to start, these motions prepare your joints for more challenging exercises later; they also allow you to do a simple self-assessment of your range of motion and pain-free zones. With all passive/active range-of-motion exercises, never exceed or force your current range of motion. Do not use medication to mask pain.

PENDULUM (FORWARD AND BACKWARD)

SHOULDER

GOAL: increase range of flexion and extension

STARTING POSITION: Place your unaffected arm on a table or other stable surface for support, and lean over.

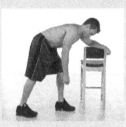

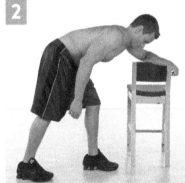

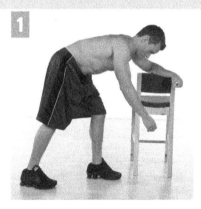

1–2. Gently swing your affected arm back and forth several times along the side of your body. Use your shoulder muscles, rather than your arm, to pull the arm down.

3. If you experience no pain, gradually increase the swings.

Switch sides and repeat.

VARIATION: For additional traction, hold a dumbbell.

PENDULUM (ACROSS BODY)

GOAL: increase range of adduction and abduction

STARTING POSITION: Place your unaffected arm on a table or other stable surface for support, and lean over.

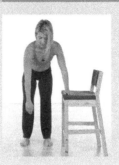

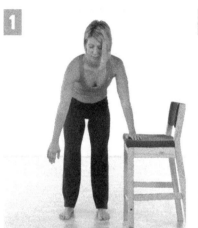

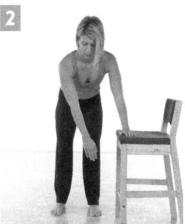

1–2. Gently swing your affected arm right and left several times across your body. Use your shoulder muscles, rather than your arm, to pull the arm down.

3. If you experience no pain, gradually increase the width of your swings.

Switch sides and repeat.

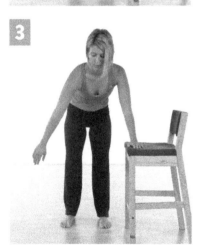

VARIATION: For additional traction, hold a dumbbell.

HANGING ARM CIRCLES	SHOULDER

GOAL: increase general range of motion

STARTING POSITION: Place your unaffected arm on a table or other stable surface for support, and lean over.

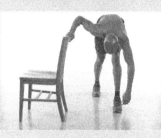

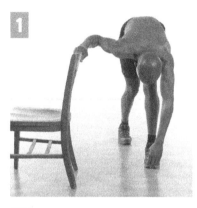

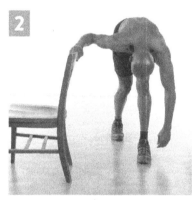

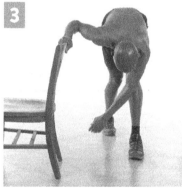

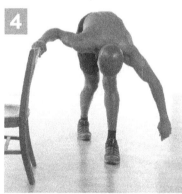

1–2. Gently swing your affected arm several times in a small, clockwise direction. Use your shoulder muscles, rather than your arm, to pull the arm down.

3–4. If you experience no pain, gradually increase circle size.

Gently swing your arm in a small, counterclockwise direction, then switch sides and repeat.

SHOULDER BOX   TRAPEZIUS

GOAL: increase flexibility and prepare shoulder for sports play

STARTING POSITION: Stand tall with proper posture.

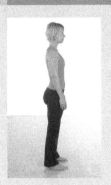

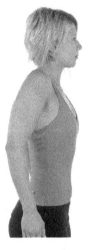

1

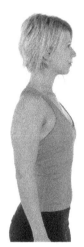

2

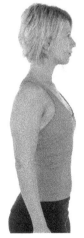

3

1. Inhaling deeply through your nose, slowly shrug your shoulders up to your ears.

2. Pull your shoulders back and squeeze the shoulder blades together and down.

3. Exhaling through your mouth, lower your shoulders and return to starting position.

Repeat as desired.

SHOULDER ROLLS

TRAPEZIUS

GOAL: warm up the shoulder joint

STARTING POSITION: Sit with proper posture in a stable chair. Inhale slowly and deeply through your nose.

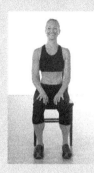

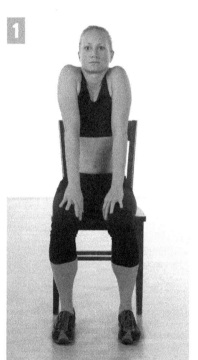

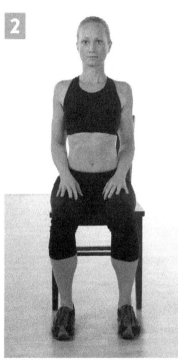

1. Roll your shoulders forward, attempting to touch your shoulders together.

2. Squeeze your shoulder blades together, moving your shoulders back and opening your chest.

Repeat as desired.

VARIATION: You can also perform the exercise while standing with proper posture.

ELBOW TOUCHES

GOAL: warm up the shoulder joint

STARTING POSITION: Sit with proper posture in a stable chair. Place your left hand on your left shoulder and your right hand on your right shoulder.

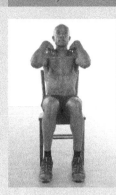

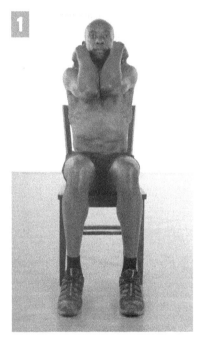

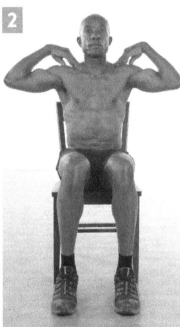

1. Slowly bring your elbows together in front of your body.

2. Bring your elbows out to the side while squeezing your shoulder blades together. Hold for a moment, focusing on opening up your chest.

Return your elbows to starting position.

Repeat as desired.

VARIATION: Perform while standing with proper posture.

PEC STRETCH

SHOULDER, CHEST

GOAL: increase shoulder girdle flexibility

STARTING POSITION: Sit with proper posture in a stable chair. Clasp your hands behind your head.

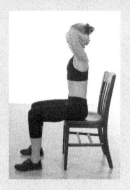

1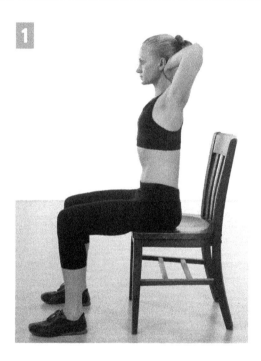

1. Slowly move your elbows backward while squeezing your shoulder blades together. Focus on opening up your chest and tightening your upper-back muscles. Only go as far back as is comfortable and hold for a moment.

Return to starting position.

Repeat as desired.

VARIATION: A partner can help you increase the stretch by gently and slowly taking your elbows back. Use extreme caution when performing partner stretches.

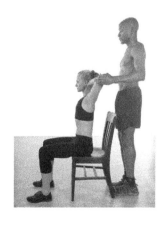

APPLE PICKERS

DELTOIDS

GOAL: increase shoulder mobility

STARTING POSITION: Stand tall with proper posture and place your left hand on your left shoulder and your right hand on your right shoulder.

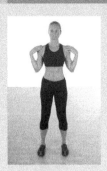

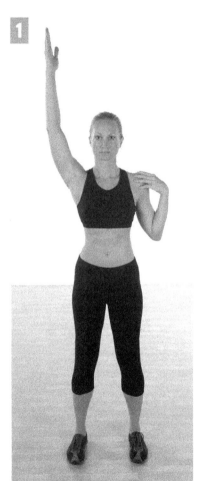

1

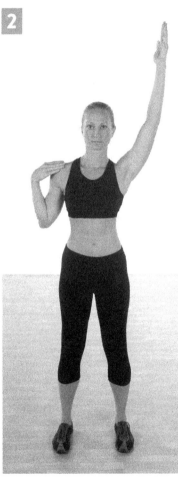

2

1. Move your right hand up to the ceiling.

2. Place your right hand back on your right shoulder and move your left hand up to the ceiling.

Continue alternating sides.

PICTURE FRAME	SHOULDER

GOAL: increase mobility

STARTING POSITION: Stand with proper posture. Place your right hand on your left elbow and your left hand on your right elbow.

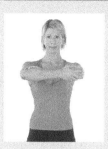

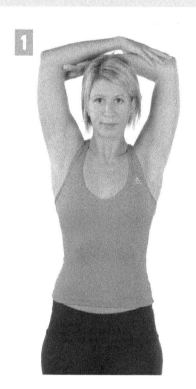

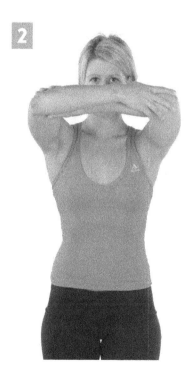

1. Slowly raise your arms overhead, lifting your arms no higher than your comfort level; make sure not to arch your back. Hold the position for a moment. You are now framing your face in a picture frame created by your arms—smile.

2. Return to starting position.

Repeat as desired.

VARIATION: This can also be performed while sitting with proper posture in a stable chair.

TABLE REACH

SHOULDER

GOAL: increase range of motion

STARTING POSITION: Sit with proper posture at a table and place your affected arm on the table.

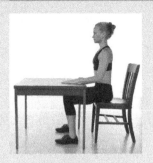

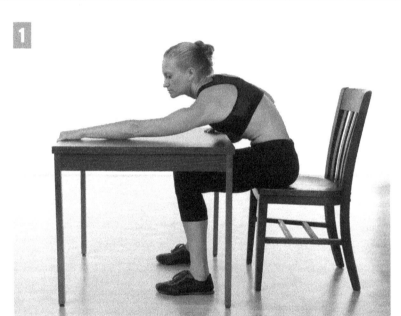

1. Slowly slide your arm forward across the table as if reaching toward the other side.

Switch sides and repeat.

CHOKER

ROTATOR CUFF

GOAL: increase range of motion

STARTING POSITION: Sit with proper posture in a stable chair.

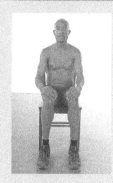

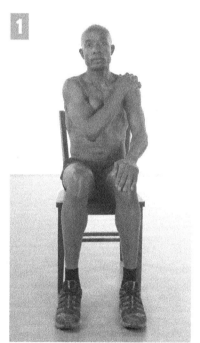

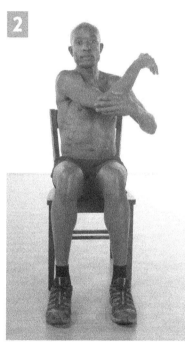

1. Place your right hand on your left shoulder.

2. Place your left hand on your right elbow and gently press your right elbow toward your throat. Your elbow should be in line with your nose. Hold for a moment.

Switch sides and repeat.

VARIATION: Perform while standing with proper posture.

OVER THE TOP

GOAL: increase flexibility

STARTING POSITION: Sit with proper posture in a stable chair.

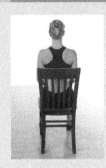

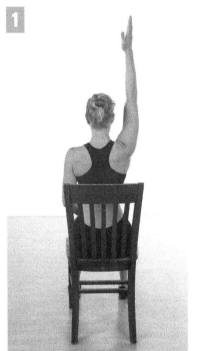

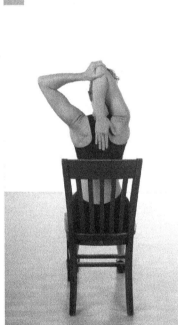

1. Reach your right hand up to the ceiling.

2. Bend your arm and let your forearm rest against the back of your head. Place your left hand on your right elbow and gently press your right arm down your back as far as feels comfortable. Hold for a moment.

Switch sides and repeat.

VARIATION: Perform while standing with proper posture.

INTERNAL ROTATION STRETCH

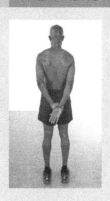

GOAL: increase range of internal rotation

STARTING POSITION: Stand tall with proper posture and place both arms behind your back. Grab your affected arm's wrist with the unaffected arm.

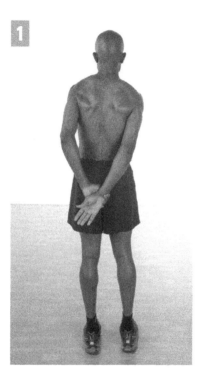

1 **1.** Gently push the affected arm up the spine. Do not force it!

ARM PULLS

GOAL: provide gentle traction

STARTING POSITION: Stand tall with proper posture. Place a soft pad against your ribs, between your affected arm and torso. Place your affected arm in front of your body and grasp your affected wrist with your unaffected hand.

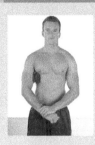

1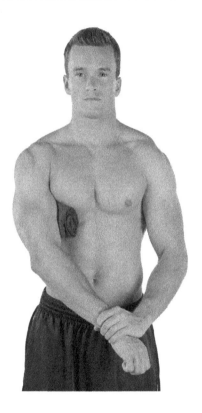

1. Gently pull your arm down and across your body. Hold for 5–10 seconds.

Repeat as desired.

VARIATION: You can also try the arm pull by taking your affected arm behind your back.

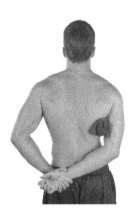

TABLE STRETCH

GOAL: open up shoulder girdle

NOTE: This is a controversial exercise. Consult your doctor before attempting.

STARTING POSITION: Stand with your back against a solid table and place both palms on the edge of the table. If you feel discomfort, STOP!

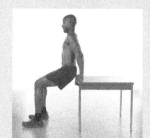

1

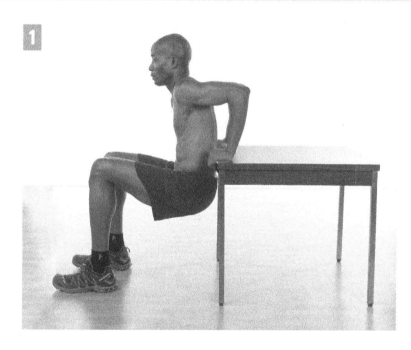

1. Bending your knees, slowly lower your buttocks towards the floor to enhance the stretch. Only go as far as feels comfortable—do not force it!

Return to starting position.

ACTIVE RANGE OF MOTION SERIES

Each exercise in this advanced series is performed while standing, with focus on range of motion and shoulder blade stabilization. Many of the standing exercises using exercise bands can be performed in a pool. Water exercise provides the advantage of resistance in both directions, and it is difficult to apply too much downward-force load. Once your strength improves, try increasing resistance by using aqua-gloves or hand paddles.

ANGELS

SHOULDER

GOAL: increase range of motion and muscle tone

STARTING POSITION: Stand tall with proper posture and your arms at your sides, palms facing forward.

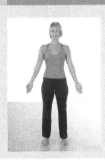

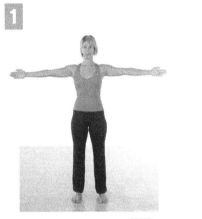

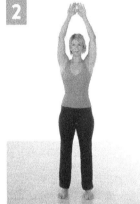

1–2. Inhale deeply through your nose and slowly raise your arms out to the sides as high as comfortably possible. Try to touch your thumbs above your head.

3. Exhale through your mouth and slowly lower your arms.

Repeat as desired.

VARIATION: Turn palms up.

ADVANCED: Try this movement with your back and arms against a wall.

SOUP CAN POURS

DELTOIDS, ROTATOR CUFF

GOAL: increase shoulder flexibility

STARTING POSITION: Stand tall with proper posture and your arms at your side, palms facing backward.

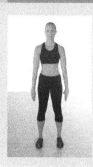

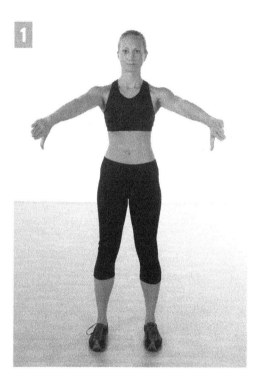

1. Inhale deeply through your nose and bring both arms slightly forward (roughly 45 degrees). As you raise your arms out to the sides, keep your palms facing backward, actively rotating your thumbs down. Raise your arms no higher than shoulder height.

Exhale through your mouth as you lower your arms.

Repeat as desired.

VARIATION: For an additional challenge, try this with dumbbells.

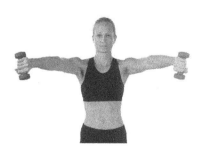

UPPER-BACK STRETCH

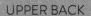

UPPER BACK

GOAL: stretch upper-back muscles

STARTING POSITION: Stand tall with proper posture and clasp your hands in front of your body.

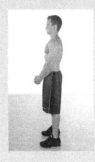

1

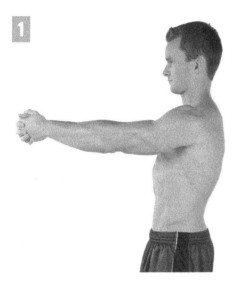

1. Straighten your arms and slowly lift them to shoulder height.

2. Once at approximately shoulder height, turn your palms forward and hold the stretch for 5–15 seconds.

Return to starting position.

ADVANCED: Slowly move your arms to the left and right.

2

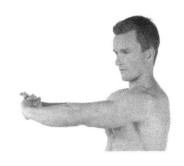

THE WAVE

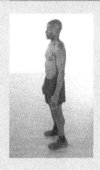

GOAL: increase range of flexion

STARTING POSITION: Stand tall with proper posture and your arms alongside your body.

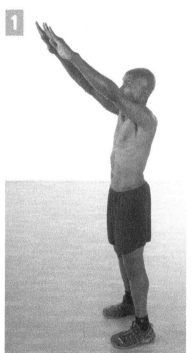

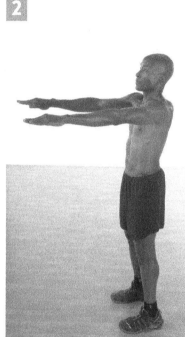

1. Keeping your palms down, raise your arms to a comfortable height, aiming for a complete range of motion.

2. Once at a desired height, slowly lower your arms.

VARIATION: Turn thumbs upward.

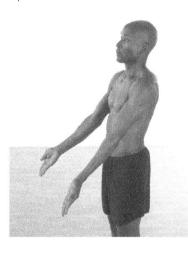

SHOULDER BLADE PINCH

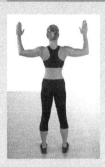

GOAL: improve posture and muscles

STARTING POSITION: Stand tall with proper posture. Raise your arms up to shoulder height and bend your elbows 90 degrees so that your fingers point to the ceiling.

1

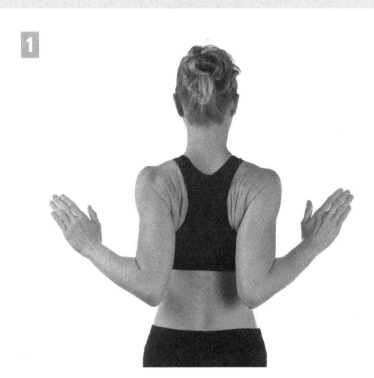

1. Lower your elbows toward your buttocks, as if you're trying to put them in your back pockets. Hold for 5–10 seconds. Do not hold your breath. The purpose of this exercise is to open up your chest and contract the muscles of the upper back, keeping your shoulders back and down.

WOOD CHOPS | SHOULDER

GOAL: increase and improve range of shoulder flexion and functional shoulder movements

STARTING POSITION: Stand tall with proper posture. Clasp your hands in front of your body.

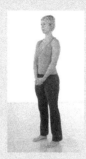

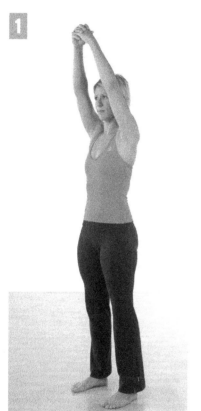

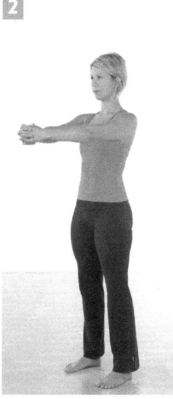

1. Keeping your arms straight, slowly raise them as high as possible. Do not arch your back.

2. Slowly lower your arms to starting position.

VARIATION: For a slight challenge, keep your hands separated as you lower and raise them.

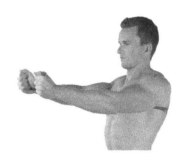

CONDOR

GOAL: increase range of motion, stabilization, and rhythm of the scapular and humerus joint

STARTING POSITION: Stand tall with proper posture.

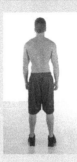

1. Slowly lift your arms to shoulder height and extend your arms out to the sides, keeping your shoulder blades down and inward.

2. Pinch your shoulder blades together.

Slowly lower your arms to starting position.

| RESCUE ME | SCAPULAR AND HUMERUS JOINTS |

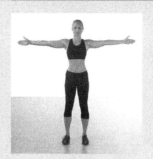

GOAL: increase scapular/humerus rhythm

STARTING POSITION: Stand tall with proper posture. Raise both arms out to the sides to make a T shape, palms facing forward.

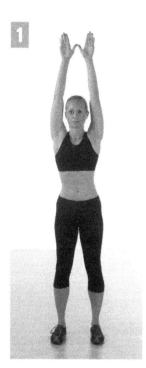

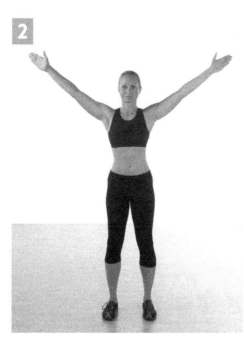

1. From the T position, attempt to keep your shoulder blades down and in "locked position." Raise your arms straight above your head if possible. This resembles the motion of a drowning victim signaling for help.

2. Lower your arms to T position, focusing on shoulder blade placement.

TOUCH DOWN

SHOULDER

GOAL: increase range of flexion

STARTING POSITION: Stand tall with proper posture and your arms alongside your body.

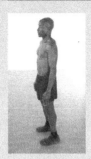

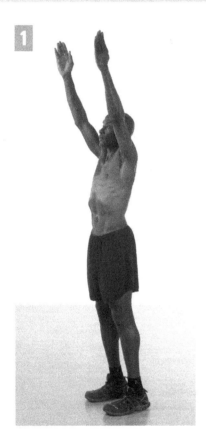

1

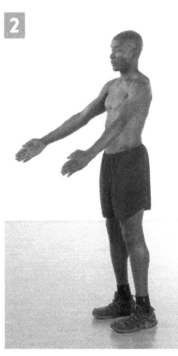

2

1. Turn your thumbs up while keeping your arms straight, and raise your arms as high as possible.

2. Lower your arms slowly.

VARIATION: Perform the same movement, except focus on keeping your shoulder blades down and in. You'll notice that you have less shoulder flexibility, but that is okay.

PUSH BACKS

GOAL: increase extension of the shoulder girdle and posterior muscle tone

STARTING POSITION: Stand tall with proper posture and your arms alongside your body.

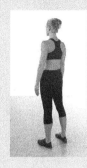

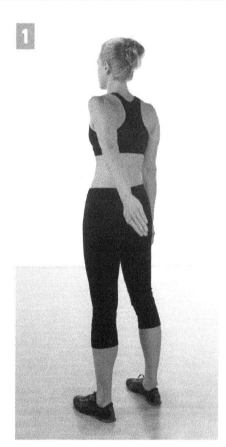

1. Slowly and carefully move one arm back as far as is comfortable. Hold for 3–5 seconds. If you feel pain, do not continue.

Slowly return to starting position and switch sides. Compare the range of motion between your affected arm and unaffected arm.

THE ZIPPER

GOAL: increase flexibility

STARTING POSITION: Stand tall with proper posture. Raise your right arm above your head and let your hand drop behind your neck.

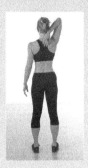

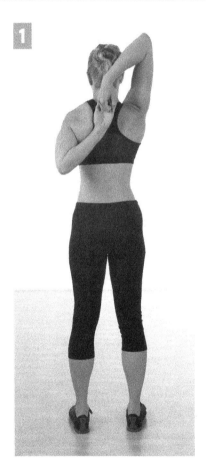

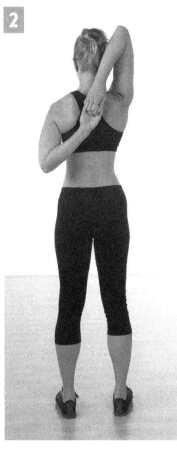

1. Bring your left hand behind your back and clasp the fingers of your right hand.

2. Gently pull down your right hand with your left hand. Hold the position for a comfortable moment.

Switch sides and repeat.

VARIATION: If you cannot reach your hands, use a towel.

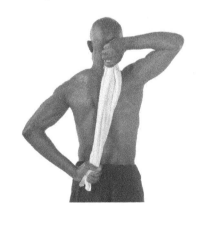

ROTATOR CUFF (EXTERNAL ROTATION)

DELTOIDS, ROTATOR CUFF

GOAL: increase rotator cuff strength

STARTING POSITION: Stand tall with proper posture and your arms at your sides. Place a rolled-up towel between your arm and your torso. Bend your affected elbow 90 degrees so that your thumb points up.

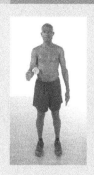

1

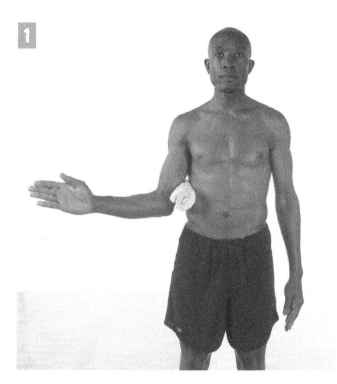

1. Keeping your elbow as close to your body as possible and your forearm parallel to the floor, rotate your forearm out to the side.

Rotate your forearm back in toward your body. Repeat as desired before switching sides.

VARIATION: Try this with your palm facing down or up.

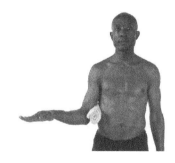

FLOOR SERIES

This series of exercises can be done on the floor or in your bed.

ELBOW TOUCHES (SUPINE)

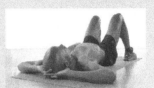

GOAL: increase range of shoulder motion, stretch chest muscles, strengthen upper-back muscles

STARTING POSITION: Lie on your back, bend your knees, and place your feet on the floor/bed. Clasp your hands behind your head.

1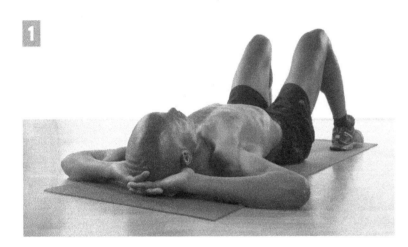

1. Gently press your elbows toward the floor or bed while squeezing your shoulder blades together. Stay within a comfortable pain zone; you'll feel a stretching sensation in the chest area. Hold for 2–5 seconds.

FINGER CIRCLES

GOAL: increase range of motion

STARTING POSITION: Lie on your back, bend your knees and place your feet on the floor/bed. Extend your affected arm up toward the ceiling, palm facing inward.

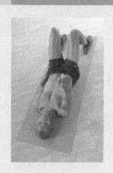

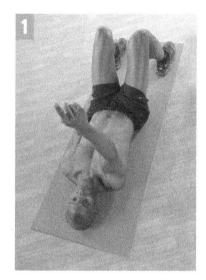

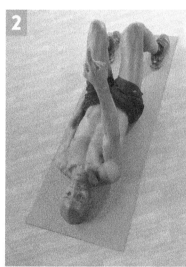

1–3. Slowly move your arm in small circles, as if you're drawing circles on the ceiling with your fingers. Draw your shoulder blades as close together as is comfortable.

Increase the size of the circle and then reverse directions.

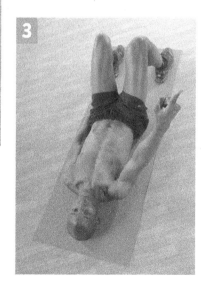

STRAIGHT-ARM STRETCH

GOAL: increase range of motion and flexibility of shoulder girdle

STARTING POSITION: Lie on your back, bend your knees, and place your feet on the floor/bed. Extend your affected arm toward the ceiling with your thumb pointing back and palm facing inward. Try to retract your shoulder blades together and keep them glued to the floor.

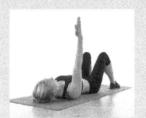

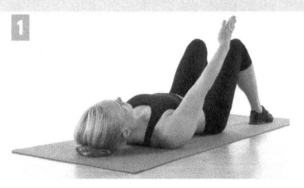

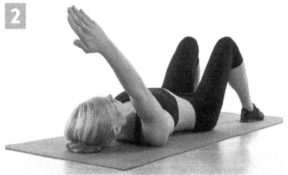

1–2. Keeping your arm straight the entire time, slowly move your pinky down next to your body, then slowly extend your arm back over your head, attempting to get your thumb comfortably close to the floor. Don't force the motion in either direction.

3–4. Repeat the movement, attempting to increase your range each time.

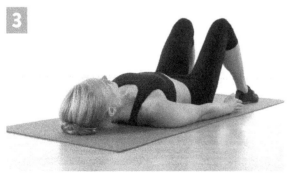

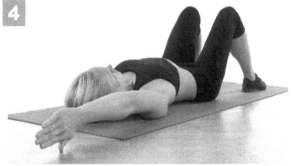

I'S, Y'S, AND T'S

GOAL: increase range of motion

STARTING POSITION: Lie on your back, bend your knees, and place your feet on the floor or bed to keep your back in neutral position. Raise both arms toward the ceiling, palms facing inward.

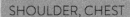
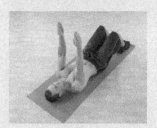

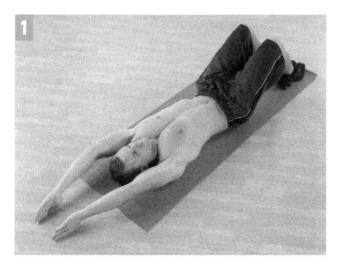

1. Keeping your back flat, slowly take both arms directly backward, staying within your comfortable range of motion. From a top view, your arms will look like an "I" formation.

2. Return to starting position.

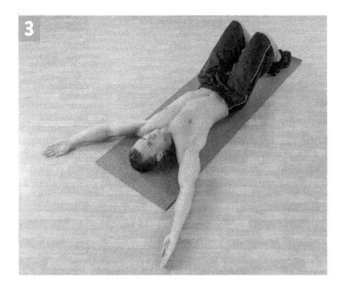

3. Now take both arms back and slightly out to the sides at a 45-degree angle, forming a "Y" shape.

4. Return to starting position.

5. Now slowly open both arms directly to the sides to form a "T" shape.

Return to starting position.

CROSSING GUARD

ROTATOR CUFF

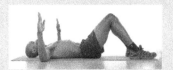

GOAL: increase external rotation

STARTING POSITION: Lie on your back, bend your knees and place your feet on the floor/bed. Rest your elbows on the floor/bed. Bend your arms 90 degrees so that your forearms are perpendicular to your body and your fingers are pointing towards the ceiling, palms facing forward.

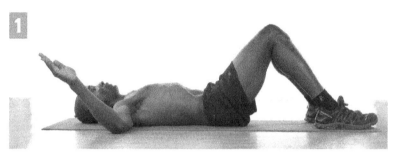

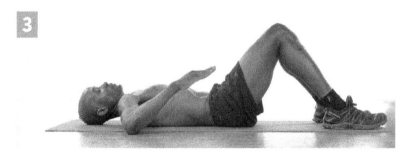

1–2. Slowly allow the backs of your hands to drop towards the floor. Caution: Most people are very tight in this region—stay within your comfort zone.

3. Slowly bring the palms of your hands forward to the floor.

Return to starting position.

EXTERNAL ROTATION (SUPINE)

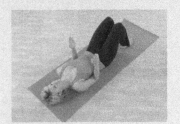

GOAL: increase external rotation, strengthen rotator cuff

STARTING POSITION: Lie on your back, bend your knees, and place your feet on the floor/bed. Rest your elbows on the floor. Bend your arms 90 degrees so that your forearms are perpendicular to your body and your fingers are pointing toward the ceiling, palms facing inward.

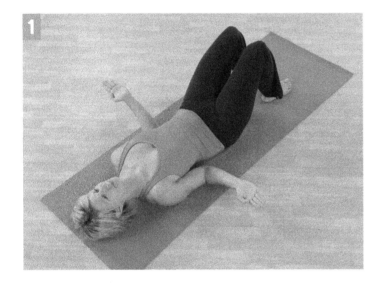

1. Slowly allow the backs of your hands to drop toward the floor. Caution: Most people are inflexible in this region. Don't force it—stay within your comfort zone.

Return to starting position.

VARIATION: For an additional challenge, hold the ends of a band in each hand.

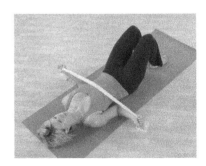

INTERNAL ROTATION (SUPINE)

ROTATOR CUFF

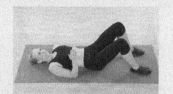

GOAL: increase internal rotation, strengthen rotator cuff muscles

STARTING POSITION: Lie on your back, bend your knees, and place your feet on the floor/bed. Rest your elbows on the floor. Bend your arms 90 degrees so that your forearms are perpendicular to your body and your fingers point toward the ceiling, palms facing inward.

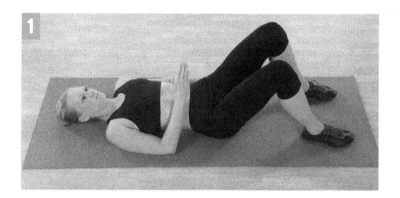

1. Keeping your elbows on the floor, slowly allow the palms of your hands to drop inward toward your belly button. Don't force it—be sure to stay within a comfortable zone.

Return to starting position.

INTERNAL ROTATION (SIDE-LYING)

ROTATOR CUFF

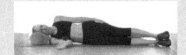

GOAL: increase internal rotation

STARTING POSITION: Lie on your affected side with your elbow against your torso and the back of your hand on the floor/bed. Bend your arm so that your forearm is perpendicular to your body. You may want to place a small, rolled-up towel against your ribs. If it is uncomfortable to lie on your affected side, avoid this exercise or perform it on a soft surface.

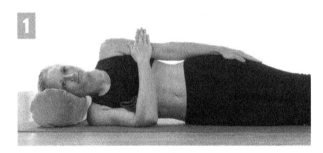

1. Slowly lift your fist up toward your belly.

Return to starting position.

Repeat, then switch sides.

VARIATION: For an additional challenge, try holding a dumbbell.

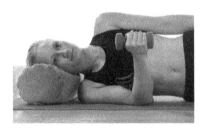

EXTERNAL ROTATION (SIDE-LYING)

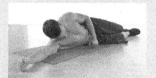

GOAL: increase external rotation

STARTING POSITION: Lie on your unaffected side. Rest your affected elbow on your rib cage, with your arm bent in an L position; make a fist. Your palm will face the floor. You may want to place a small, rolled-up towel between your torso and your elbow.

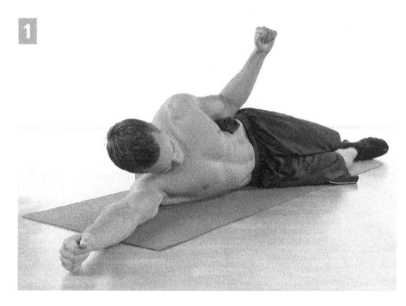

1. Slowly lift your fist up and back as high as possible. Don't force it or move rapidly.

Return to starting position.

Repeat, then switch sides.

VARIATION: For an additional challenge, try holding a dumbbell.

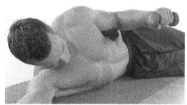

SHOULDER BLADE PUSH-UP

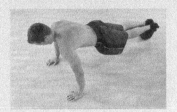

GOAL: stabilize shoulder blades

STARTING POSITION: Assume a push-up position either on your knees or toes, keeping a nice line from the top of your head to your feet.

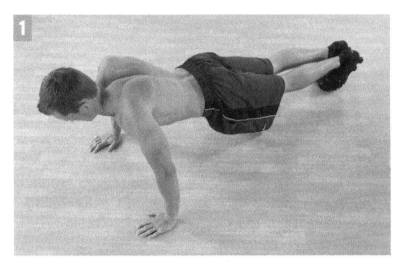

1. While in push-up position, contract the muscle that pulls your shoulder blades together. Hold for 5–10 seconds.

Release and relax.

VARIATION: To reduce the weight in your arms, try this from your knees or by leaning against a countertop.

NOTE: This is a more challenging exercise and should be introduced with caution.

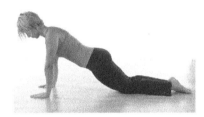

CANE/STICK SERIES

To assist your affected arm, this series of exercises uses a stick, cane, or belt. The purpose of these exercises is to maintain or improve range of motion.

SUPINE PRESS

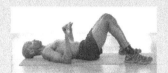

GOAL: foster range of motion

STARTING POSITION: Lie on your back, bend your knees, and place your feet on the floor. Grasp the stick or cane with each hand, shoulder-width apart, so that the stick is above your chest. Keep your elbows on the floor, close to your body.

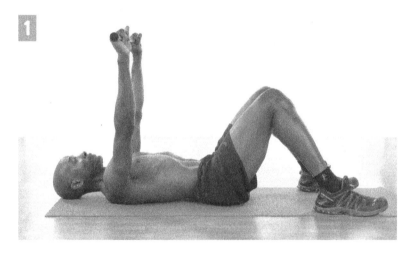

1. Press the stick up toward the ceiling until both arms are fully extended.

Return to starting position.

VARIATION: To make the exercise harder, try draping a sandbag weight across the stick. Use caution; secure the sandbag weight so it does not fall off and hit you.

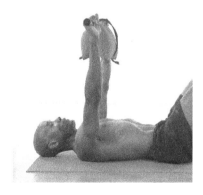

PULL-OVERS

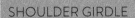
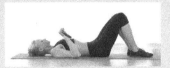

GOAL: foster range of motion

STARTING POSITION: Lie on your back, bend your knees, and place your feet on the floor. Grasp the stick or cane with each hand, shoulder-width apart, so that the stick rests across your chest.

1

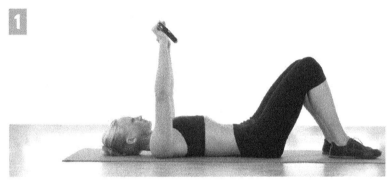

1. Press the stick up toward the ceiling until both arms are fully extended.

2. Keeping your arms straight, slowly lower the stick behind your head and toward the floor. Do not force it!

2

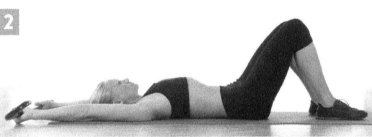

3. Return to center.

VARIATION: To make the exercise harder, try draping a sandbag weight across the stick. Use caution; secure the sandbag weight so it does not fall off and hit you.

3

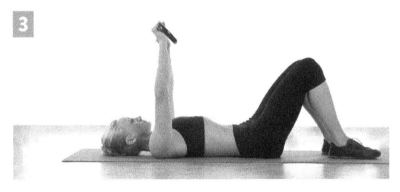

LATERAL DROPS

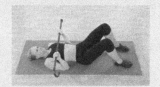

GOAL: foster range of motion

STARTING POSITION: Lie on your back, bend your knees, and place your feet on the floor. Grasp the stick or cane with each hand, shoulder-width apart, so that the stick rests across your chest.

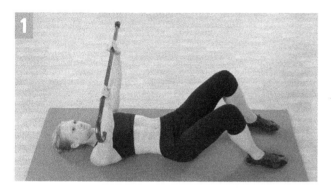

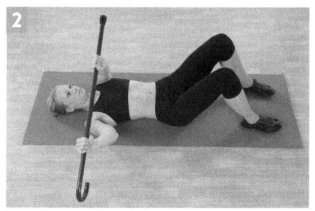

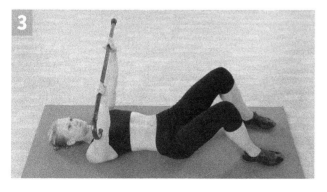

1. Press the stick up toward the ceiling until both arms are fully extended.

2. Keeping your arms as straight as possible and your shoulder blades close to your spine, slowly lower the stick to the right side as far as you comfortably can. Try to keep both shoulders on the floor

3. Return to center and "reset" your shoulder blades (pull your shoulder blades back to gently push your chest upward).

Repeat on the other side.

REVERSE LIFT

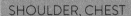

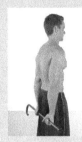

GOAL: increase range of motion

STARTING POSITION: Stand tall with proper posture. Grasp a strap, stick, or cane behind your buttocks with your hands shoulder-width apart.

1

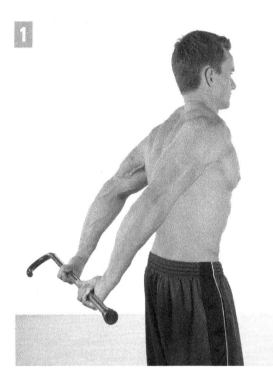

1. Keeping your arms straight, attempt to lift them away from your body. Focus on squeezing your shoulder blades together. Hold this position for as long as it's comfortable.

Return to starting position.

NOTE: This is a more challenging exercise and should be introduced with caution.

ADVANCED: Instead of using a device, interlock your hands behind your back and perform the movement.

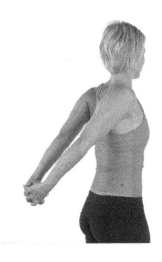

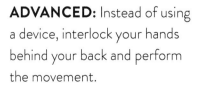

STICK PRESS

GOAL: increase range of motion and improve shoulder strength

STARTING POSITION: Stand tall with proper posture. With both hands, hold the stick or cane against your chest at shoulder height, palms facing forward.

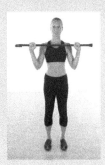

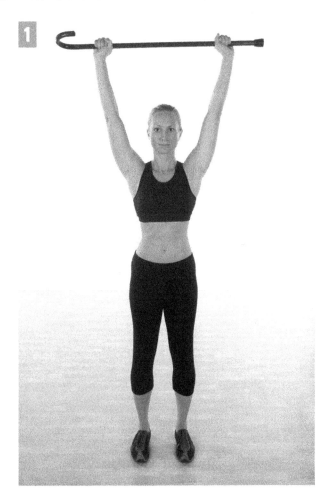

1. Press the stick up toward the ceiling as high as you comfortably can. Avoid arching your back to increase the height. If keeping your arms straight stresses your joints too much, you can press up with your arms angled.

Return to starting position.

NOTE: This is a more challenging exercise and should be introduced with caution.

VARIATION: This exercise can also be performed while seated and/or with a sandbag weight draped across the stick or cane.

BACK SCRATCH

GOAL: increase internal range of motion

STARTING POSITION: Stand tall with proper posture, and hold on to the cane or stick with both hands behind your buttocks.

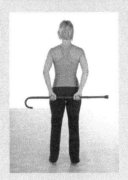

1

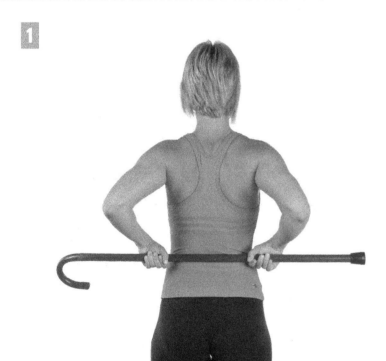

1. Slowly raise the stick up your back as if spinning a rolling pin up your back. Imagine squeezing a pencil between your shoulder blades. If you are extremely inflexible, do not perform this exercise until you are pain free or receive medical clearance.

Return to starting position.

NOTE: This is a more challenging exercise and should be introduced with caution.

ROLLER SERIES

This section utilizes the foam roller. The basic premise of a foam roller is to loosen the facia, a type of connective tissue. By applying pressure to the area of greatest restriction, circulation can be improved and restrictions released. Researchers found that rolling over the area for 30 to 60 seconds provided the best benefit. It is a method of self-massage.

The foam roller provides an unstable surface that will challenge the stabilizer muscles of the body more than if you were to do the exercises without the prop. These exercises should only be done when you are symptom free and looking to challenge yourself. Please note: It is generally agreed not to roll over soft areas of the body like your belly. If you have postural hypertension, balance issues, or difficulty getting up and down from the floor, avoid the roller series.

First, you'll need to safely lie on a roller. Here's how you do it:

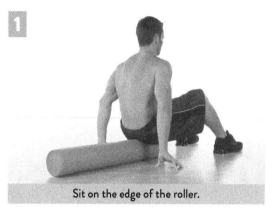

Sit on the edge of the roller.

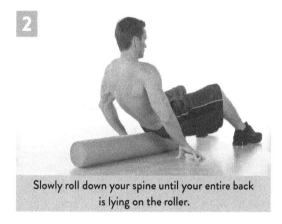

Slowly roll down your spine until your entire back is lying on the roller.

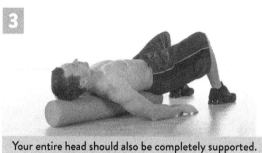

Your entire head should also be completely supported.

WINDMILLS ON ROLLER

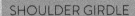

SHOULDER GIRDLE

GOAL: increase range of motion and stabilization of shoulder

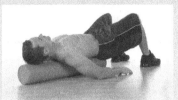

STARTING POSITION: Lie on a foam roller, resting your head and the entire length of your back on it. Bend your knees and place your feet on the floor; place your arms on the floor alongside your body for balance. Breathe naturally and allow adequate time for your chest and shoulder region to relax and open up. For many people, this is an adequate stretch and it's okay to stop here without progressing to the following steps.

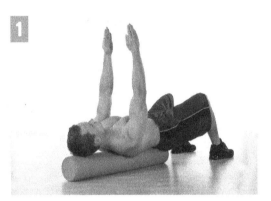

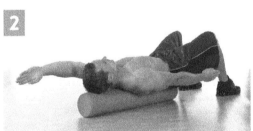

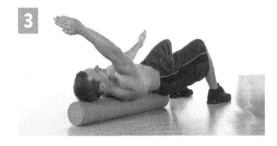

1. Once comfortable and stable, extend both arms up to the ceiling while maintaining balance on the roller; your palms should face each other. Be sure to stabilize your core the entire time by contracting your abs.

2. Allow one arm to move forward and the other backward. Stay within your comfortable range of motion.

3. Reverse direction.

Release and relax.

ELBOW DROPS

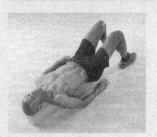

GOAL: open chest and shoulder girdle

STARTING POSITION: Lie on a foam roller, resting your head and the entire length of your back on it. Bend your knees and place your feet on the floor; place your arms on the floor alongside your body for balance. Breathe naturally and allow adequate time for your chest and shoulder area to relax and open up. For many people, this is an adequate enough stretch and it's okay to stop here without progressing to the following steps.

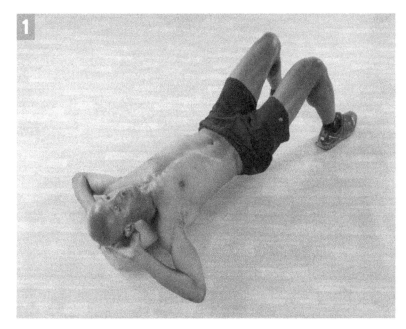

1. Once comfortable, place your hands under your head and slowly allow your elbows to "drop" toward the floor. You should not expect to touch the floor. Stop if this is uncomfortable. Hold the stretch while breathing naturally.

Release and relax.

SHOULDER SLAPS

GOAL: realign the shoulder girdle

STARTING POSITION: Lie on a foam roller, resting your head and the entire length of your back on it. Bend your knees and place your feet on the floor; extend your arms up to the ceiling, palms facing each other.

SHOULDER GIRDLE

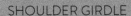
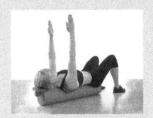

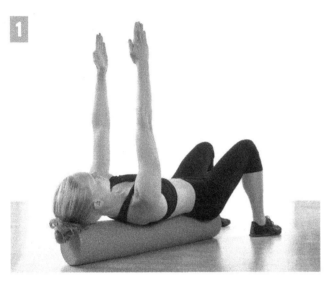

1. Reach your fingers up to the ceiling, allowing your shoulder blades to come off the roller.

2. Keeping your arms straight, completely relax your shoulder muscles, allowing your shoulder blades to "slap" back down on the roller.

Repeat as desired.

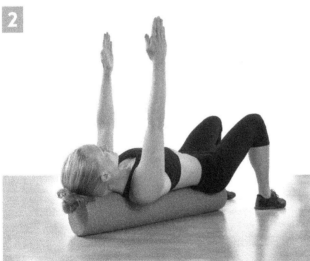

I'S, Y'S, AND T'S ON ROLLER

GOAL: increase shoulder flexibility and stabilization

CAUTION: This is an advanced exercise. Do not do this exercise until you have completed the I's, Y's, and T's (page 85) on a solid surface.

STARTING POSITION: Lie on a foam roller, resting your head and the entire length of your back on it. Bend your knees and place your feet on the floor; place your arms on the floor alongside your body for balance. Breathe naturally and allow adequate time for your chest and shoulder area to relax and open up. Focus on opening up the shoulder girdle and keeping your shoulders back. For many people, this is an adequate enough stretch and it's okay to stop here without progressing to the following steps.

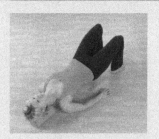

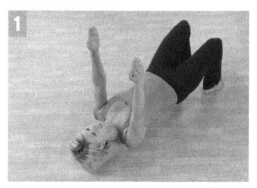

1. Once comfortable, extend both arms up toward the ceiling.

2. Now move both arms directly back and forth, making an "I," while focusing on shoulder blade stabilization.

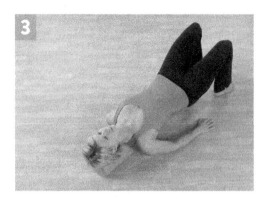

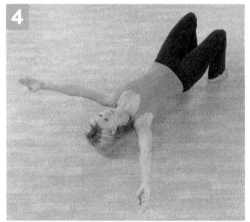

3. Relax in starting position.

4. After completing the I's, take both arms slightly back and out to the sides at a 45-degree angle, forming a "Y" shape.

5. Relax in starting position.

6. After completing the Y's, slowly open both arms directly to the sides to form a "T" shape.

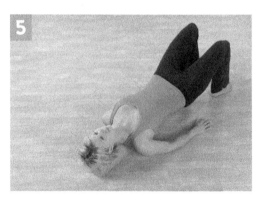

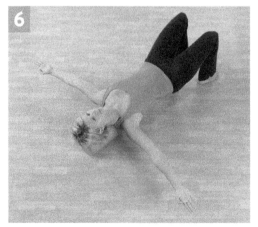

WALL/DOOR SERIES

This series of exercises utilizes a door, doorframe, table, or wall as a support prop to facilitate the activity. Never hold your breath when performing static exercises.

FINGER WALKING (FORWARD)

SHOULDER

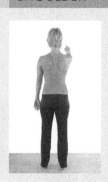

GOAL: increase flexion

STARTING POSITION: Face a wall and stand an arm's length away from it. Reach with the fingertips of your affected arm to touch the wall at shoulder height.

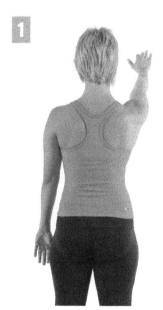

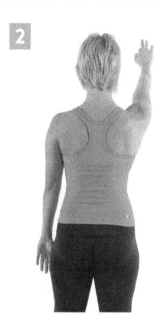

1–2. Slowly walk your fingers up the wall as high as you comfortably can. Do not arch your back or twist your body to gain height.

Return to starting position. Switch sides and repeat.

NOTE: Never force the elbows or arms into an uncomfortable zone! Avoid extreme stretching positions.

FINGER WALKING (SIDE)   SHOULDER

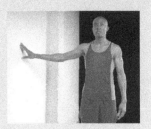

GOAL: increase abduction

STARTING POSITION: Using your affected shoulder, stand sideways to a wall that is an arm's length away. Reach with your fingertips to touch the wall just below shoulder level.

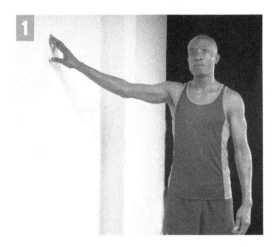

1–2. Slowly allow your fingers to walk up the wall as high as you comfortably can. Never exceed your comfortable range of motion. Do not lean or elevate your shoulder to gain additional height.

Return to starting position. Switch sides and repeat.

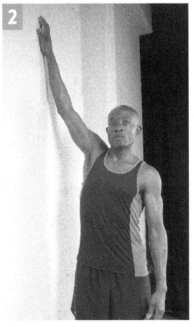

SIDE CLOCK

SHOULDER

GOAL: increase flexion/extension

STARTING POSITION: Using your affected shoulder, stand sideways to a wall that is an arm's length away. Stretch your affected arm straight up the wall (12 o'clock position).

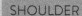
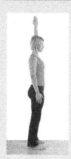

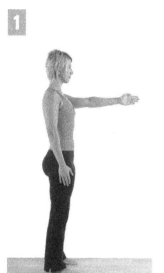

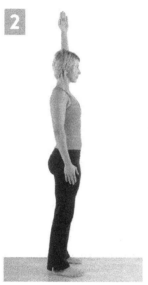

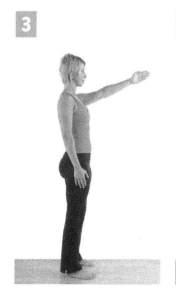

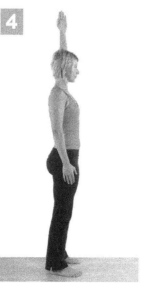

1. Slowly move your arm down the wall to the 3 o'clock position.

2. Return to 12 o'clock.

3. Slowly move to the 2 o'clock. Do not force it if you're inflexible!

4. Return to starting position.

Switch sides and repeat. Your arm will now point to the 9, 12, and 10 o'clock positions.

WALL CIRCLES

SHOULDER

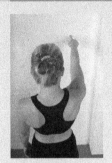

GOAL: increase circumduction/rotation

STARTING POSITION: Face a wall and stand an arm's length away from it. Touch the wall with the index finger of your affected arm.

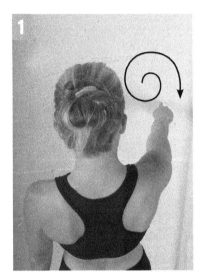

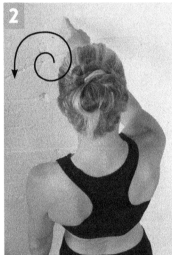

1–2. Slowly draw a small circle clockwise. If comfortable, make increasingly larger circles.

Reverse directions, making the circles progressively smaller. Switch sides and repeat.

CORNER STRETCH

CHEST, SHOULDER (ADVANCED)

GOAL: increase chest and shoulder flexibility

STARTING POSITION: Start with your spine along the edge of a wall's corner. Focus on keeping your lower back and head against the corner. Breathe naturally.

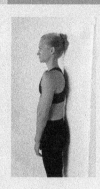

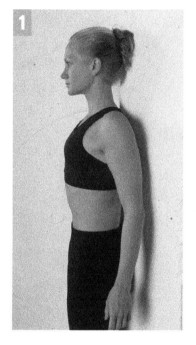

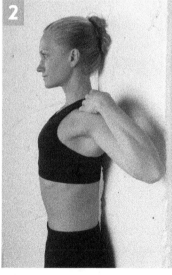

1. Slowly allow your shoulder blades to wrap around the corner with the goal of opening up the chest area. Hold for 5–10 seconds.

2. If possible, place your hands on your shoulders and gently enhance the stretch by pulling your elbows back with the muscles of your upper back. Hold for 5–10 seconds. If this is uncomfortable, do not force it.

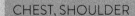

CHEST STRETCH (DOORWAY)

CHEST, SHOULDER

GOAL: increase shoulder flexibility

STARTING POSITION: Stand in the middle of a doorframe. Place your hands on each side of the doorframe at a comfortable height.

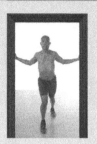

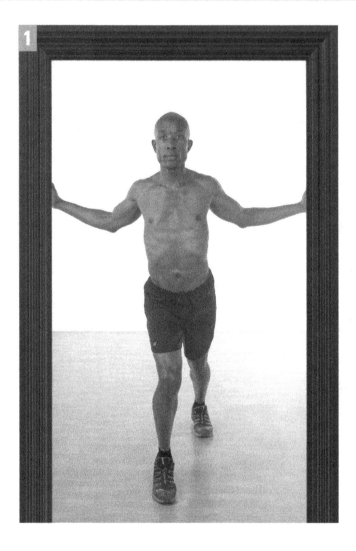

1 Slowly lean forward, allowing your body weight to stretch the front of your shoulders. Never exceed your comfortable range of motion. Hold for 20–30 seconds.

VARIATION: If a doorway is not available, ask a partner to grab your wrists and gently pull your arms behind you.

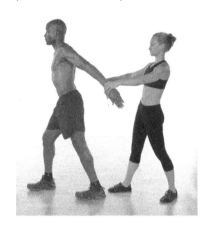

STICK UP

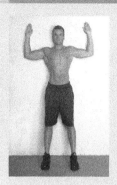

GOAL: open up chest and shoulder region, and tone functional shoulder muscle

STARTING POSITION: Stand with your back and head against the wall.

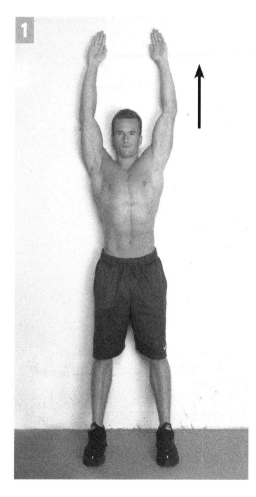

1. Bend your arms 90 degrees, placing the backs of your hands on the wall. Hold for 3–5 seconds.

Slowly raise your arms up along the wall, keeping your back and head close to the wall. This exercise is very difficult for some people—do not force it!

ELBOW TOUCHES (AGAINST WALL)

PECTORALS

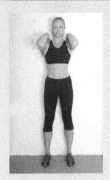

GOAL: increase shoulder girdle flexibility

STARTING POSITION: Stand with your back and head against the wall. Place your hands on your shoulders and point your elbows forward.

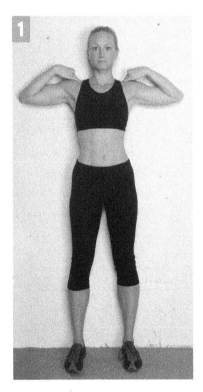

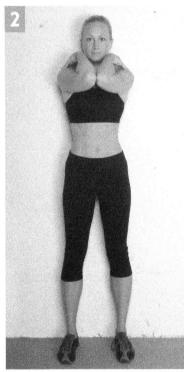

1. Carefully move your elbows toward the wall. Don't arch your back to increase your range. Touching the wall is not critical—the goal is to feel a gentle stretch in your chest and shoulders. Don't force it!

2. Slowly move your elbows back to center until you can touch them together.

Return to starting position.

DOUBLE-HAND PRESS

UPPER BACK

GOAL: increase strength in upper back

STARTING POSITION: Stand with your back and head against the wall and your arms along your sides. Place your palms on the wall.

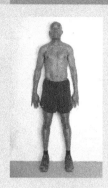

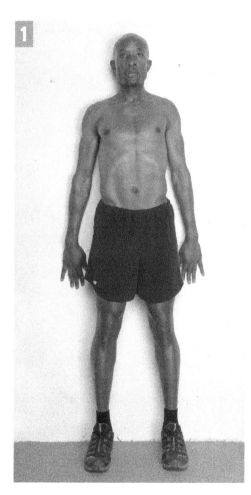

1. Gently press your hands against the wall, feeling the muscles between your shoulder blades contract. Do not hold your breath or arch your back.

WALL REACH

GOAL: passively stretch shoulder

STARTING POSITION: Stand against the edge of a wall and extend your affected arm along it. Feel the stretch through the shoulder area, and relax and breathe freely.

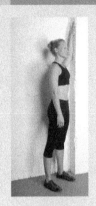

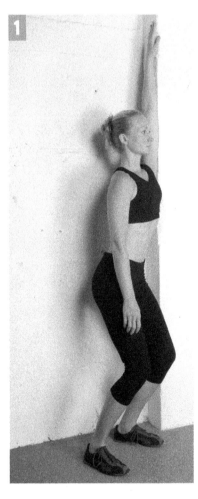

1. To enhance the stretch, slightly bend your knees to lower your body. Never exceed your comfortable range of motion.

VARIATION: This can also be done against a doorframe.

EXTERNAL ROTATION (WALL)

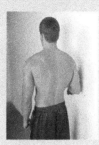

GOAL: increase external rotation strength

STARTING POSITION: Stand against a wall. Bend the elbow of your affected arm 90 degrees, keeping your elbow positioned next to your ribs. Place the back of your affected hand against the wall. Place a small pillow between your arm and torso.

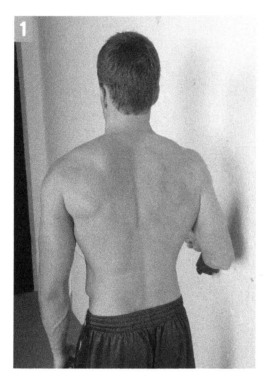

1 Press the back of your hand into the wall and hold 3–5 seconds. This is a very subtle isometric movement.

VARIATION: This can also be done against a doorframe.

INTERNAL ROTATION (DOOR)

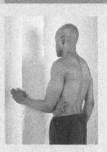

GOAL: increase internal rotation strength

STARTING POSITION: Stand facing the edge of a wall or a doorframe. Bend the elbow of your affected arm 90 degrees, keeping your elbow positioned next to your ribs. Place the palm of your hand against the doorframe. Place a small pillow between your arm and torso.

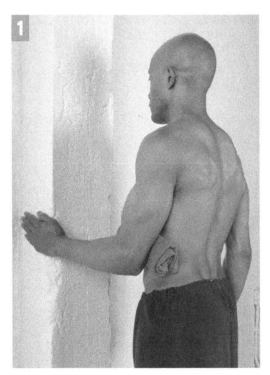

1. Press your palm into the doorframe and hold 3–5 seconds.

WALL PUSH-UP

UPPER BACK

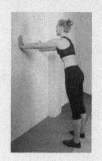

GOAL: increase stabilization of shoulder girdle

STARTING POSITION: Stand 2–3 feet away from a wall and place your palms on it, approximately chest height and shoulder-width apart.

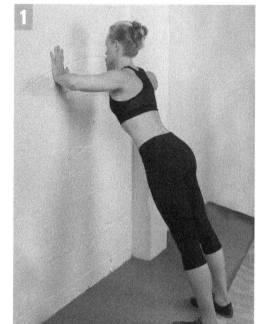

1. Slowly lower your chest toward the wall by bending your elbows. Move slowly and focus on squeezing your shoulder blades together.

Return to starting position very slowly.

VARIATION: To reduce the impact on your shoulders, you can move just your scapulas, squeezing them together and then expanding them.

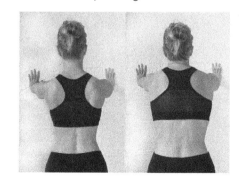

ISOMETRIC SHOULDER BLADE SQUEEZE | UPPER BACK

GOAL: increase stabilization of shoulder girdle

STARTING POSITION: Stand 2–3 feet away from a wall and place your palms on it, approximately chest height and shoulder-width apart.

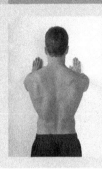

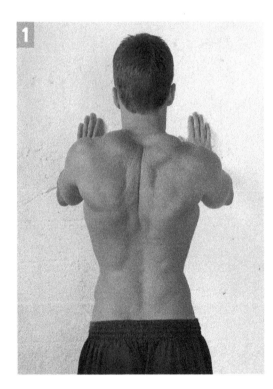

1. Slowly contract/squeeze the muscles between your shoulder blades and hold for 3–5 seconds.

ISOMETRIC FRONTAL LIFT · SHOULDER

GOAL: increase shoulder flexion strength

STARTING POSITION: Stand facing a wall and place the back of your affected hand against it.

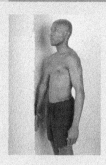

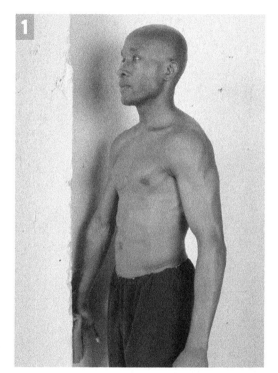

1. Press the back of your hand against the wall. Your arm should be fully extended. Hold for 3–5 seconds, utilizing enough tension to foster muscle tone.

Switch sides and repeat.

ISOMETRIC REAR LIFT

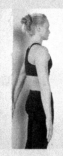

GOAL: increase shoulder extension strength

STARTING POSITION: Stand with your back to a wall.

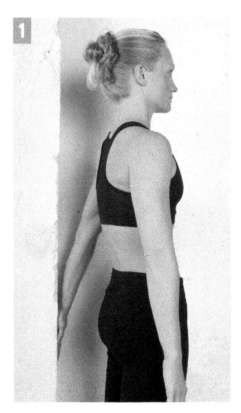

1. Press the palm of your affected hand against the wall. Hold for 3–5 seconds, utilizing enough tension to foster muscle tone.

Switch sides and repeat.

STATIC PEC STRETCH

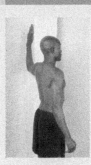

GOAL: increase shoulder extension strength

STARTING POSITION: Stand against a doorframe or the edge of a wall. Bend your elbow 90 degrees and place your forearm and hand on the wall/doorframe.

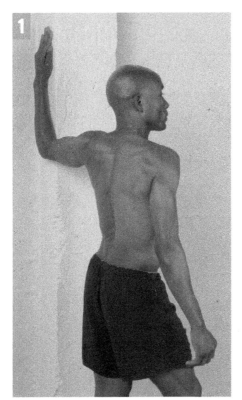

1. Slowly take a step forward, feeling the stretch in your chest.

Switch sides and repeat.

RESISTANCE CONDITIONING SERIES

This section utilizes exercise bands or handheld weights that help improve the strength and muscle tone of the shoulder girdle. Select a band that is relatively easy or flexible. Generally, the color of the band denotes the resistance level (e.g., yellow = easiest, red = medium, blue or black = hardest), but the resistance levels are not equal for all vendors. When performing strength training for habilitation purposes, do not overstrain your muscles.

Your goal should target proper form and execution. It's important, when using resistance, that you control the movement—don't allow the resistance to control you. Slowly perform the movement in both directions at the same pace (i.e., up, 2, 3, 4, hold; down, 2, 3, 4, hold). This will usually prevent further injury. For a more comprehensive menu of resistance band exercise, see *The Resistance Band Workbook* and *Injury Rehab with Resistance Bands*.

Hand position and placement is critical when using bands. Grips can be purchased, but this simple device shown below is inexpensive and quite comfortable. To make a grip, purchase a PVC pipe from any hardware store. You'll also need an exercise band. Bands with handles built in are readily available at most sporting goods stores. Once you have both, follow the steps below:

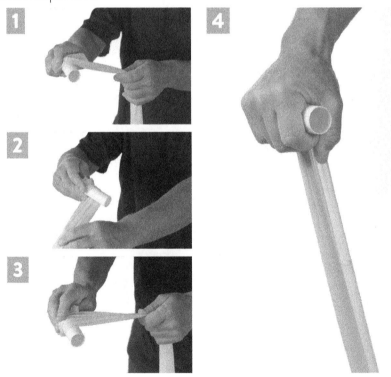

These exercises are designed to strengthen and progressively challenge the shoulder region. Being overly zealous can be hazardous to your shoulder rehab. Start slow, with the least amount of resistance, and progress with caution. There is no shame in starting very easy (this is a rehab program, not a body-building program). Never exceed safe range of motion, and ensure the bands are securely attached.

FRONTAL RAISES

DELTOIDS

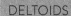

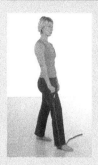

GOAL: increase shoulder flexion strength

STARTING POSITION: Stand tall with proper posture. Place one end of the band under the foot on the affected side and grasp the other end with your affected hand. Adjust the resistance by moving your hand up or down the band. Resistance should begin as you start raising your arm. Your arm should be as straight as possible but not locked.

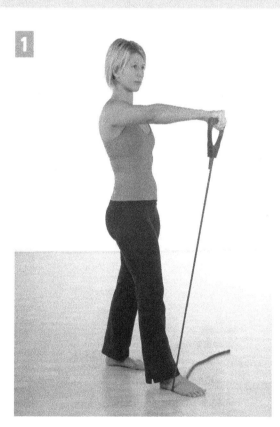

1. Slowly bring your straight arm up to shoulder height. If comfortable, raise your arm all the way up. If this is uncomfortable, lower your arm to starting position.

Switch sides and repeat.

LATERAL RAISES

GOAL: increase shoulder abduction strength

STARTING POSITION: Stand tall with proper posture. Place one end of the band under the foot of the affected side and grasp the band with your affected hand, palm down.

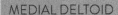

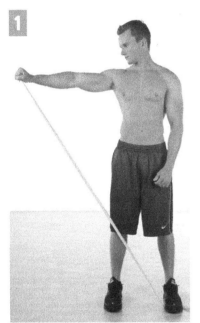

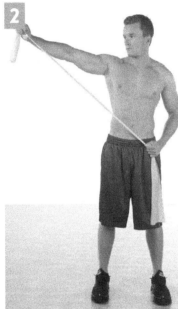

1. Slowly raise your arm out to the side until it's shoulder height. If this is uncomfortable, move the position of your arm to a different angle to find a comfort zone. If this is still uncomfortable, don't do this movement.

2. Slowly return to starting position.

Switch sides and repeat.

VARIATIONS: If you have trouble lifting your arm laterally, try taking your arm 45 degrees forward.

This exercise can also be done with dumbbell weights instead.

SHOULDER EXTENSION

GOAL: increase shoulder extension strength

STANDING POSITION: Stand tall with proper posture. Place one end of the band under the foot of the affected side and grasp the band with your affected hand, thumb pointing forward.

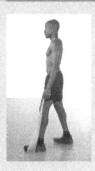

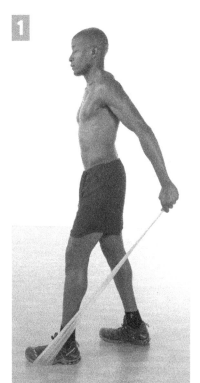

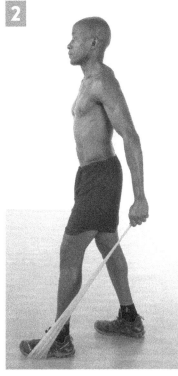

1. Slowly move your arm backward, keeping your arm straight.

2. Return to starting position.

Switch sides and repeat.

VARIATION: This exercise can also be done with dumbbell weights.

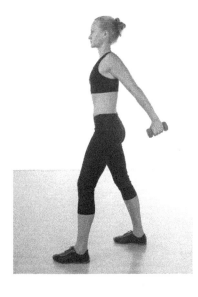

REVERSE FLY WITH BAND

SHOULDER

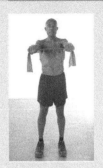

GOAL: strengthen muscles behind the shoulder blades, improve posture, provide stabilization

STARTING POSITION: Stand tall with proper posture. Grasp the exercise band in front of you with your hands shoulder-width apart and palms down. Do not wrap the band around your hands. Keeping your arms straight, raise them to approximately shoulder height.

1

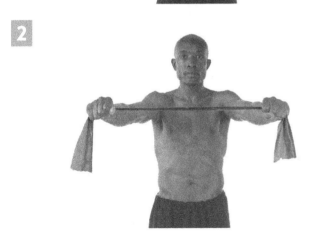

2

1. Slowly open your arms to the sides, with special focus on squeezing the muscles that bring your shoulder blades together.

2. Slowly return to starting position.

DOWNWARD SWORD FIGHTER

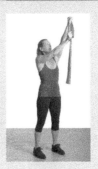

GOAL: to foster improved posture

STARTING POSITION: Stand with proper posture and hold one side of the band in your left hand slightly above your head with your thumb pointing down.

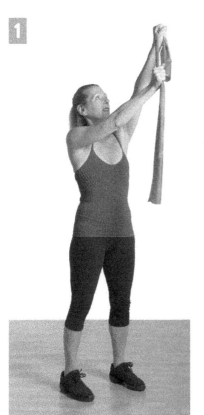

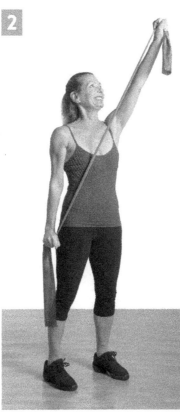

1. Grasp the band with your right hand at a location that provides adequate resistance.

2. Slowly pull your right hand diagonally down past your right hip. Slowly allow the band to return to starting position.

Repeat, then switch sides.

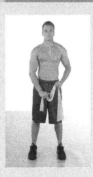

GOAL: increase upper-shoulder and back strength

STARTING POSITION: Stand tall with proper posture and hold the band with the unaffected hand. Grasp the band with the affected hand at a position that provides mild resistance.

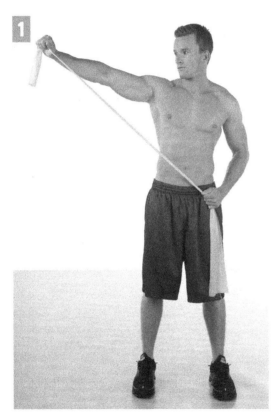

1. Keeping your unaffected arm in place, use your affected hand to pull the band diagonally up and across your body, as if pulling a sword out of its sheath.

Slowly return to starting position. Switch sides and repeat.

BIKE PUMP

GOAL: foster improved shoulder stability

STARTING POSITION: Stand with proper posture. Drape the band over your right shoulder and secure it in place with your left hand. With your right hand, grab the band at a location that provides ideal resistance. Once the band is in place, lean over slightly as if pushing down on a bike pump.

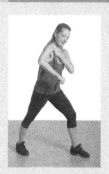

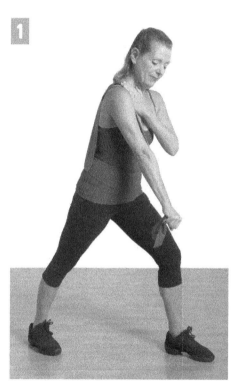

1. Slowly press your right arm down.

Slowly return to starting position. Repeat, then switch sides.

HORIZONTAL TRICEPS EXTENSION

TRICEPS / SHOULDER STABILIZATION

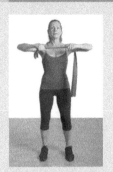

GOAL: Improve triceps tone; improve posture and shoulder stabilization when done with shoulders retracted

STARTING POSITION: Sit or stand with proper posture and grasp the band with both hands approximately shoulder-width apart and at chest height. Lift your elbows out to the sides, keeping your arms parallel to the floor.

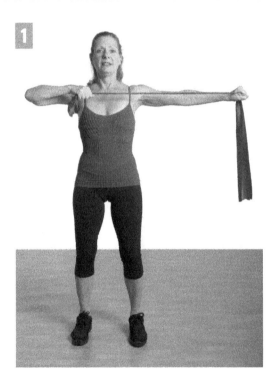

1. Keeping your right hand in place, slowly extend your left arm out to the side.

Slowly return to starting position. Repeat, then switch sides.

VARIATION: Perform the motion with both arms at the same time.

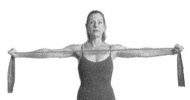

SERVING TRAY

ROTATOR CUFF

GOAL: increase rotator cuff strength

STARTING POSITION: Stand tall with proper posture. Grasp the band in both hands with your palms up. Bend both elbows 90 degrees, keeping your elbows next to your ribs.

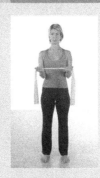

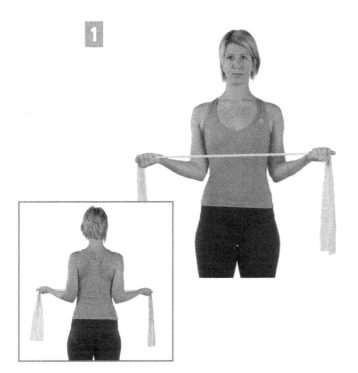

1. Keeping your elbows glued to your ribs, slowly move the ends of the band away from each other as if serving appetizers. Pinch your shoulder blades together. Hold for 3–5 seconds.

Return to starting position.

VARIATION: If you feel any discomfort, try the external rotation with band (page 133) or perform the External Rotation (Wall) (page 115).

INTERNAL ROTATION WITH BAND

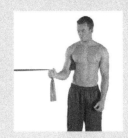

GOAL: increase internal rotation strength

STARTING POSITION: Attach the exercise band to a doorknob or a solid object (such as a heavy table leg), making sure it doesn't come loose. Position your affected side closest to the doorknob. Grasp the band with your affected hand and bend your elbow 90 degrees, placing your elbow next to your ribs. To avoid wrist pain, make sure you grasp the band correctly. You can place a rolled-up towel or small pillow between your elbow and your body.

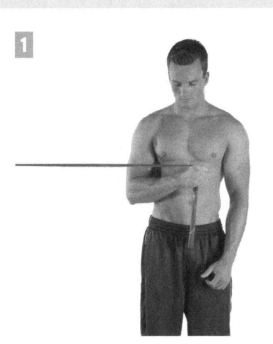

1. Keeping your elbow glued against your ribs, slowly move your hand inward, as if to place your palm on your belly button.

Slowly return to starting position. Switch sides and repeat.

VARIATIONS: If you feel any discomfort, try the Internal Rotation (Door) (page 116).

You can also do this with a partner.

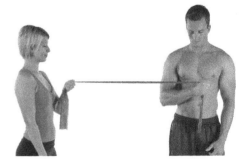

EXTERNAL ROTATION WITH BAND ROTATOR CUFF

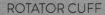
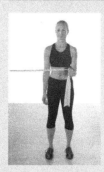

GOAL: increase external rotation strength

STARTING POSITION: Attach the exercise band to a doorknob or a solid object (such as a heavy table leg), making sure it doesn't come loose. Position your affected side farthest away from the doorknob. Grasp the band with the affected hand and bend your elbow 90 degrees, placing your elbow next to your ribs. To avoid wrist pain, make sure you grasp the band correctly. You can place a rolled-up towel or small pillow between your elbow and your body.

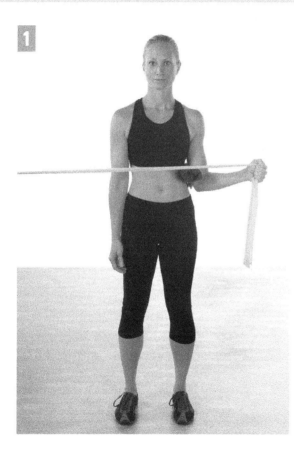

1. Keeping your elbow glued against your ribs, slowly move your hand away from the doorknob, as if opening up a coat.

Slowly return to starting position. Switch sides and repeat.

VARIATIONS: If you feel any discomfort, try the External Rotation (Wall) (page 115).

You can also have a partner hold the other end of the band.

SEATED ROWING

GOAL: increase upper-back strength

STARTING POSITION: Sit in a chair with proper posture and place a band around the foot of your affected side. Grasp the ends in each hand. Extend the leg straight forward and adjust your hands so that the band offers adequate resistance.

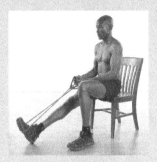

1

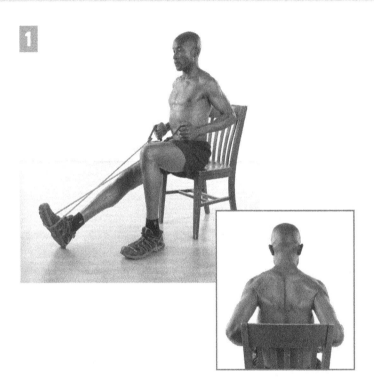

1. Slowly pull the band toward your torso, pulling your shoulder blades together and allowing your elbows to move back.

Slowly return to starting position.

PULL-DOWNS

GOAL: increase muscle strength between shoulder blades

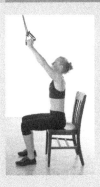

STARTING POSITION: Secure the band to the top of a door or other high, solid object. Sit in a chair with proper posture. Reach up and grab the ends of the band in each hand, making sure to grasp at a place that offers moderate resistance. Your arms will form a 45-degree angle with the door.

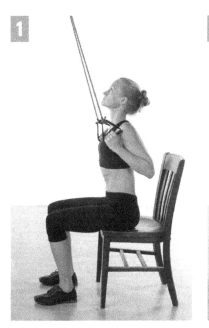

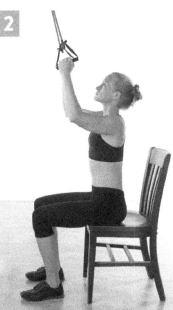

1. Slowly pull down the band toward your chest, with focus on squeezing the shoulder blades together.

2. Return to starting position while trying to keep your shoulder blades together. Only your arms should move.

BAND CHEST PRESS

CHEST, SHOULDER

GOAL: stabilize shoulder

STARTING POSITION: Stand with proper posture and place the band around your back at chest height. Grasp the ends of the band in each hand at a place that offers moderate resistance.

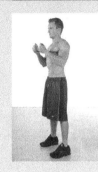

1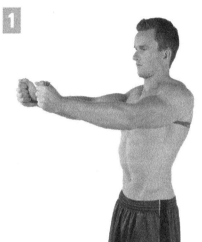

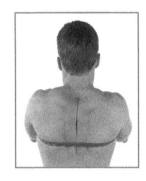

1. Fully extend your arms forward while focusing on keeping your shoulder blades back and stable.

2. Control the motion as your arms return to starting position. Do not allow the band to recoil you.

2

BAND SHOULDER PRESS

DELTOIDS

GOAL: stabilize shoulder

STARTING POSITION: Sit in a chair with proper posture and place the band around your back and under your armpits. Grasp the ends of the band in each hand at a place that offers moderate resistance.

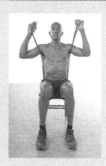

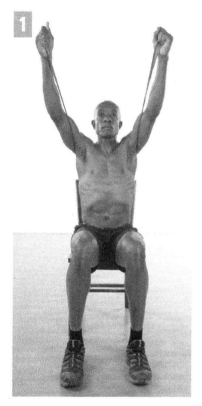

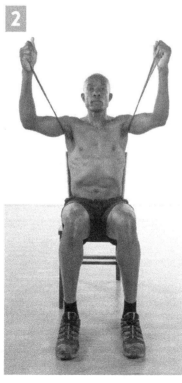

1. Fully extend your arms upward, keeping your shoulder blades together. The amount of upward motion depends on your flexibility and pain tolerance. Some people cannot go directly up and that is okay. Your focus should be on replicating the motion of putting something in an overhead luggage bin, so a slight angle is fine.

2. Control the motion as your arms return to starting position. Do not let the band recoil you.

Y'S WITH BAND	**UPPER CHEST**

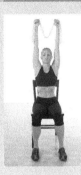

GOAL: increase shoulder girdle strength

STARTING POSITION: Sit in a chair with proper posture and grasp an end of the band in each hand, keeping your hands shoulder-width apart. Raise your arms overhead as high as is comfortable for you.

1. Keeping your head straight and squeezing your shoulder blades together, slowly pull the band apart, forming a Y with your arms.

2. Slowly return to starting position.

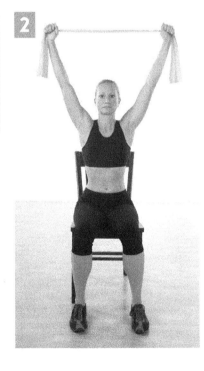

T'S WITH BAND

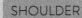

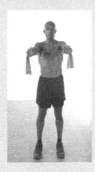

GOAL: strengthen muscles behind the shoulder blades, improve posture, provide stabilization

STARTING POSITION: Stand tall with proper posture. Grasp the exercise band in front of you with your hands shoulder-width apart and palms down. Do not wrap the band around your hands. Keeping your arms straight, raise them to approximately shoulder height.

1

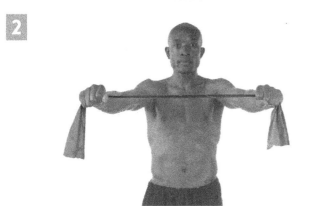

2

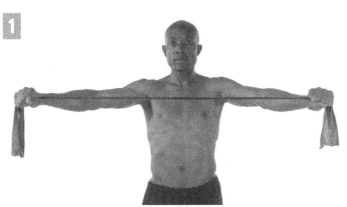

1 Slowly open your arms to the sides, with special focus on squeezing the muscles that bring your shoulder blades together.

2 Slowly return to starting position.

BAND ROLL-UPS

GOAL: improve rotation of the shoulder joint

STARTING POSITION: Sit in a chair with proper posture and hold the end of a band in one hand. Extend your arm forward at shoulder height with your thumb up.

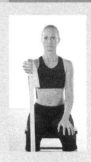

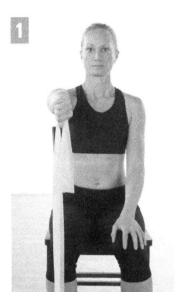

1.

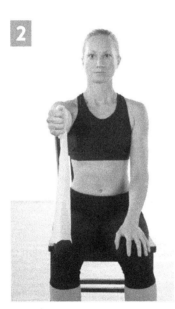

2.

1—3. Turn your hand up and down to collect the band.

Once you've rolled up the band in your hand, switch sides.

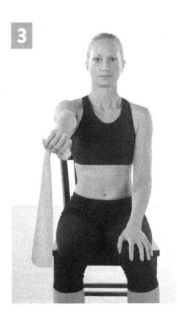

3.

SHRUG

GOAL: to condition trapezius muscle and foster improved posture

STARTING POSITION: Stand in the middle of the band with knees softly bent and grasp an end in each hand. Your hands should be in front of your hips, palms facing your body. Adjust your grip on the band until you have your desired resistance.

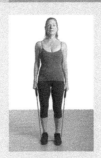

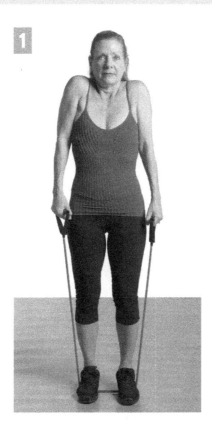

1. Keeping your arms straight, slowly "shrug" your shoulders to your ears. Hold 1–2 seconds.

Slowly return to starting position.

DUMBBELL SERIES

For the dumbbell series, never exceed a comfortable range of motion or use more weight than is comfortable. There is no shame in starting very light (these exercises are designed to rehab your injury, not as part of a body-building program).

DUMBBELL SHOULDER EXTENSION

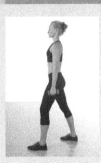

GOAL: increase rear deltoid strength

STARTING POSITION: Stand tall with proper posture and grip a dumbbell with your affected hand; you can stagger your feet if you need more balance. Your arm should be alongside your body, and your palm can face forward or backward, whichever is most comfortable.

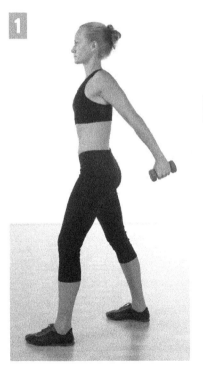

1. Keeping your arm straight, slowly move it backward, staying within your pain-free range of motion.

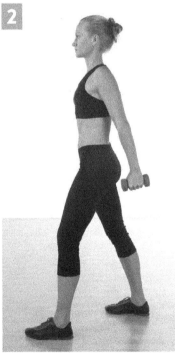

2. Slowly return your arm to starting position.

Switch sides and repeat.

VARIATION: This exercise can also be done lying face down on an incline bench.

DUMBBELL SOUP CAN POURS

GOAL: increase shoulder girdle stabilization

STARTING POSITION: Stand tall with proper posture and grip a dumbbell with your affected hand. Turn your thumb down, as if pouring out soda from a can.

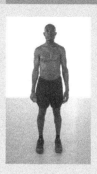

1. Slowly lift your arm out to the side at a 45-degree angle. Focus on keeping your thumb down and not moving your arm forward.

2. Lower slowly, staying within your pain-free range.

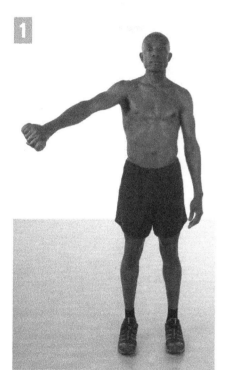

DUMBBELL REVERSE FLY

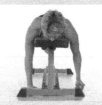

GOAL: increase upper-back strength

STARTING POSITION: Lie on your stomach on an exercise bench or bed. Let your affected arm hang off the side. Grip a dumbbell with your affected hand.

1

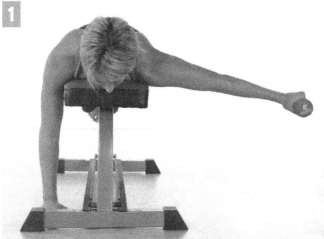

2

1. Slowly raise your arm to a parallel position with the floor.

2. Slowly return to starting position.

DUMBBELL PRESS-UP

CHEST

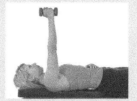

GOAL: increase shoulder girdle control

STARTING POSITION: Lie on your back on the floor or an exercise bench. Grip a dumbbell with your affected hand and lift your arm directly over your shoulder/chest. Keep your arm straight.

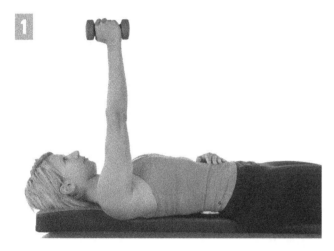

1. Keeping your arm straight, press the dumbbell up, as if trying to touch the ceiling.

2. Squeeze your shoulder blades together to return to starting position. The range of motion of this exercise is very small. If your arm is moving frequently, the exercise is not being performed correctly.

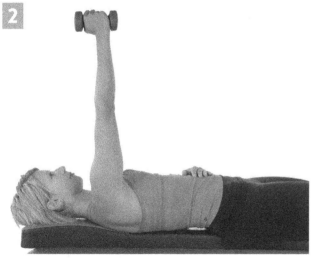

DUMBBELL SHRUGS

TRAPEZIUS

GOAL: increase shoulder girdle strength

STARTING POSITION: Stand tall with proper posture and your arms along your sides. Hold a dumbbell in each hand.

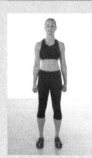

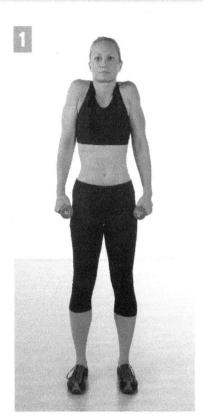

1

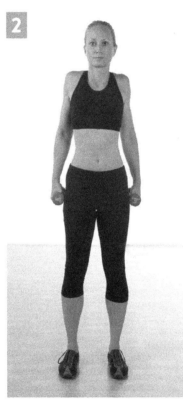

2

1–2. Shrug your shoulders up and then back, squeezing your shoulder blades together. Pretend you are making an outline of a box.

Slowly lower your shoulders to starting position.

HANGING DUMBBELL SQUEEZE

UPPER BACK

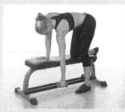

GOAL: increase upper-body strength, traction, and stabilization

STARTING POSITION: Place your right knee and hand on an exercise bench. Grip a dumbbell with your left hand and allow the weight to pull down gently on your arm. Do not use a heavy dumbbell.

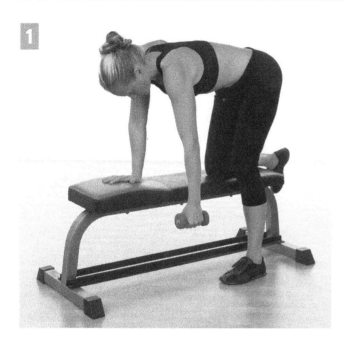

1. Keeping your arm straight, gently squeeze your shoulder blade up and back to pull the weight up. Hold for 3–5 seconds.

Slowly release and lower.

PRONE CROSSING GUARD

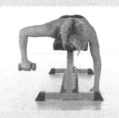

GOAL: increase strength of rotator cuff

STARTING POSITION: Lie on your stomach on a bed or an exercise bench with your affected arm hanging off the edge. Grip a dumbbell and bend your arm 90 degrees.

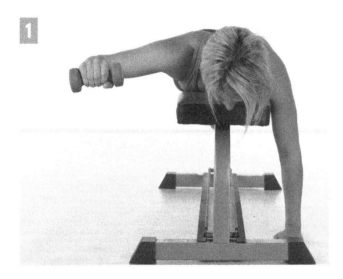

1. Keeping your elbow in place, slowly rotate your hand up to the ceiling. STOP when your hand is level with your shoulder. Many people are inflexible in this area and have limited range of motion. If you feel any discomfort, skip this exercise.

Lower your arm to starting position.

VARIATION: You can also try this with both arms simultaneously.

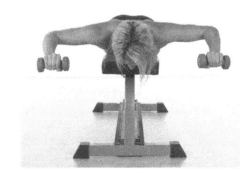

SELF-MASSAGE

The therapy ball is a wonderful self-help massage tool to reduce muscle tightness and provide deep-muscle massage and release pressure. The advantage of the therapy ball over other self-massage tools is a multi-directional massage for the area in need. It decreases soft tissue adhesions, increasing range of motion and flexibility. It also decreases muscle soreness. Self-massage is best performed when the muscle is warm. Here we use the standard tennis ball as well as the commercially available foam roller, which can be purchased online and at various local retailers, including medical suppliers, yoga/Pilates studios, and sporting goods stores. For more information, consider looking at *Trigger Point Therapy with the Foam Roller* or the *Therapy Ball Workbook*, both published by Ulysses Press. As a precaution, always consult your health professional before engaging in self-massage options.

Note: A tennis ball works fine, but some people use a golf ball while others purchase a massage ball at the sporting goods store.

TENNIS BALL METHOD 1	UPPER BACK, SHOULDER

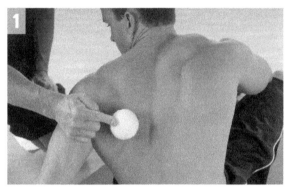

1–3. With a single tennis ball, lie on your back, placing the tennis ball under the point of discomfort to release pressure.

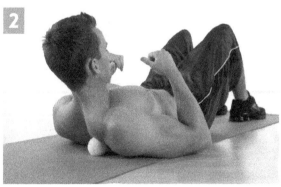

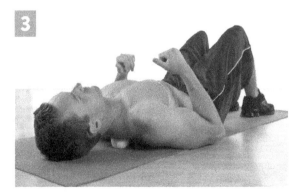

TENNIS BALL METHOD 2

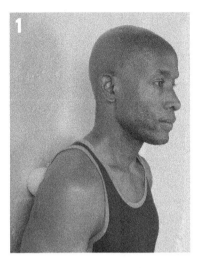 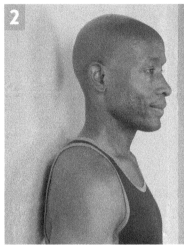

1–2. Place a tennis ball between your back and a wall and roll around to release pressure.

TENNIS BALL METHOD 3

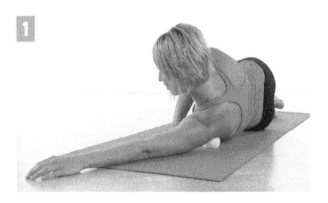

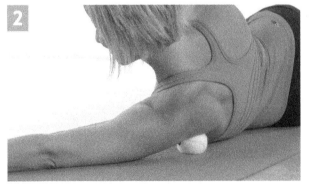

1–2. To target tight lats, lie on your side and place the tennis ball under your armpit. Roll around to release tightness.

TENNIS BALL METHOD 4 — CHEST, SHOULDER

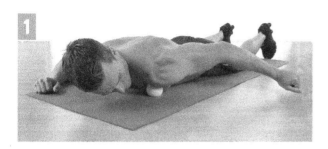

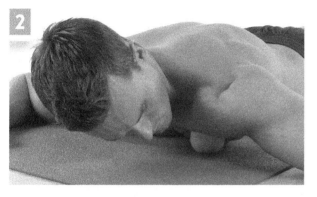

1–2. To target the front of your shoulder, lie on your front, placing the tennis ball under the point of discomfort to release pressure.

TENNIS BALL METHOD 5 — CHEST, SHOULDER

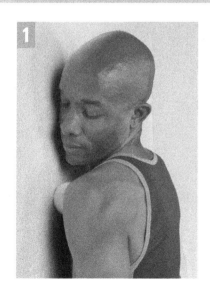

1. Place a tennis ball between the front of your shoulder and a wall and roll around to release tension.

TENNIS BALL METHOD 6 UPPER BACK

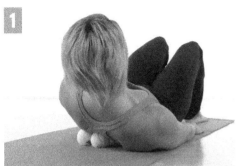

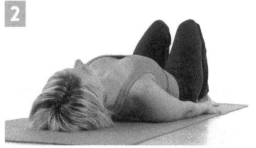

1–2. Connect two tennis balls together with tape so that they look like googly eyes. Lie on them so that they're between your shoulder blades.

TENNIS BALL METHOD 7 UPPER BACK

The nice thing about the sock is that you can more easily target those awkward areas of the back.

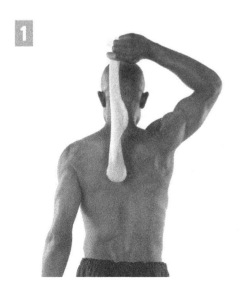

1. Take an athletic sock and place 1 or 2 tennis balls inside it. Swing the sock overhead and let it hang behind your back. Press your back and the balls against the wall, releasing tension.

FOAM ROLLER (BACK) | BACK

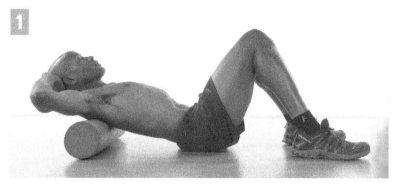

1. Sit on the floor and place your upper back on a foam roller. Clasp your hands behind your head.

2. Roll back and forth to release tension.

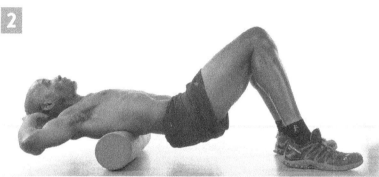

FOAM ROLLER (SIDE) — LATISSIMUS DORSI

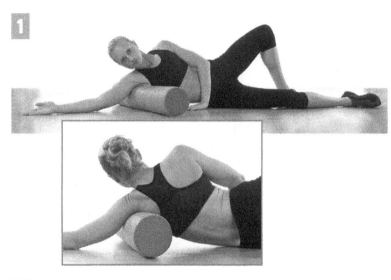

1. Lie on your side with the foam roller under your armpit.

2–3. Roll back and forth to release tension.

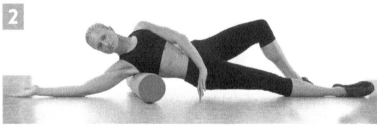

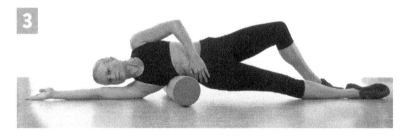

ICE

To create the cooling massage tool, place water in a paper cup and freeze it. An ice massage is best done after exercise. Practice extreme caution when using ice to avoid frostbite. Consult your health professional for the best protocol for you to use regarding the application of ice and heat and over-the-counter lotions.

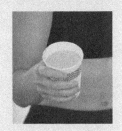

1. Peel back the paper cup as needed.

2. Apply the cup of ice on the sore spot, moving the cup around—do not leave it on one spot.

3. Ask a partner to apply the ice on the hard-to-reach places.

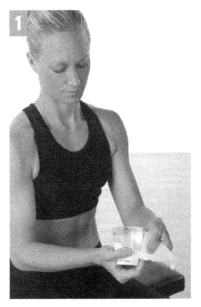

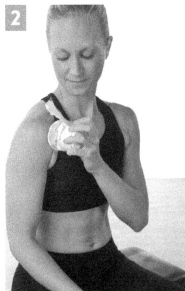

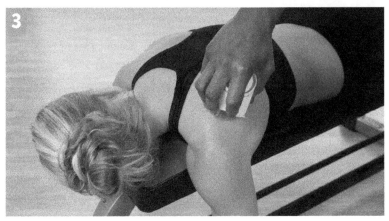

RESOURCES

American Academy of Orthopaedic Surgeons
6300 North River Road
Rosemont, IL 60018
(847) 823-7186
www.aaos.org

American Board of Orthopaedic Surgery
400 Silver Cedar Court
Chapel Hill, NC 27514
(919) 929-7103
www.abos.org

American Chronic Pain Association
P.O. Box 850
Rocklin, CA 95677
(800) 533-3231
www.theacpa.org

American Physical Therapy Association
3030 Potomac Avenue, Suite 100
Alexandria, VA 22305
(800) 999-2782
www.apta.org

Harvard Health Letter
www.health.harvard.edu/newsletters/
harvard_health_letter

Tuffs University Health Letters
www.nutritionletter.tufts.edu

Women's Health Magazine
www.womenshealthmag.com

INDEX

A

Abduction zones, 33–34
Acromioclavicular (AC) joint ligaments, 7
Acromioclavicular (AC) joints, 6
Acromion, 6
Active range of motion exercise series, 70–81
Adhesive capsulitis. *See* Frozen shoulder
Age, and shoulder dysfunction, 11
Agonist muscles, 8
Anatomy, 6–9; illustrated, 7, 9
Angels (exercise), 70
Antagonist muscles, 8
Apple Pickers (exercise), 62
Arm Pulls (exercise), 68
Arthritis, 15, 31; exercises, 51

B

Back Scratch (exercise), 98
Band Chest Press (exercise), 136
Band exercise series. *See* Resistance conditioning exercise series
Band Roll-Ups (exercise), 140
Band Shoulder Press (exercise), 137
Bands. *See* Exercise Bands
Baseball, exercise programs 44
Basketball, exercise programs 45
Benefit-to-risk ratio, 36–37, 38
Bike Pump (exercise), 129
Bones, 6; illustrated, 7

Breastbone. *See* sternum
Bursa, 8
Bursitis, 18–20; exercises, 52

C

Calcification tendinitis, 16
Cane/stick exercise series, 93–98
Cartilage, 8
Chest Stretch (Doorway) (exercise), 110
Choker (exercise), 65
Circles (exercises), 57, 83, 108
Clavicle, 6
Collar bone. *See* Clavicle
Conditioning exercise, programs, 43–44
Condor (exercise), 76
Construction jobs exercise program, 49
Controversial/inappropriate exercises, 36–39
Coracobrachialis muscles, 9
Coracoclavicular ligaments, 7
Corner Stretch (exercise), 109
Corrective exercise programs, 50–52
Crossing Guard (Basic) (exercise), 87
Crossing Guards (exercises), 87, 148
Cumulative trauma disorder. *See* Repetitive motion injuries

D

Deltoid muscles, 9
Desk jobs, exercise programs, 49

Dislocation, 14; exercises, 52

Doctor visits, 5, 11. *See also specific conditions*

Door/wall exercise series, 105–21

Do's and don'ts, 35

Double-Hand Press (exercise), 113

Downward Sword Fighter (exercise), 127

Drops (exercises), 95, 101

Dumbbell exercise series, 142–48

Dumbbell Press-Up (exercise), 145

Dumbbell Reverse Fly (exercise), 144

Dumbbell Shoulder Extension (exercise), 142

Dumbbell Shrugs (exercise), 146

Dumbbell Soup Can Pours (exercise), 143

E

Elbow Drops (exercise), 101

Elbow Touches (Against Wall) (exercise), 112

Elbow Touches (Basic) (exercise), 60

Elbow Touches (Supine) (exercise), 82

Elbow touches (exercises), 60, 82, 112

Exercise bands, 70, 122; exercise series, 122–41

Exercise programs, 40–52; conditioning, 43–44; corrective, 50–52; and safety, 42; sports-related, 44–48; work-related, 49

Exercises: active range of motion series, 70–81; cane/stick series, 93–98; floor series, 82–92; inappropriate/controversial, 36–39; passive and gentle series, 55–69; resistance conditioning series, 122–48; roller series, 99–104; self-massage series, 149–55; wall/door series, 105–21

Extension zones, 34

External Rotation (Side-Lying) (exercise), 91

External Rotation (Supine) (exercise), 88

External Rotation (Wall) (exercise), 115

External Rotation with Band (exercise), 133

External rotations (exercises), 81, 88, 91, 115, 133

F

Finger Circles (exercise), 83

Finger Walking (Forward) (exercise), 105

Finger Walking (Side) (exercise), 106

Flexion zones, 34

Floor exercise series, 82–92

Flys (exercises), 126, 144

Foam Roller (Back) (exercise), 153

Foam Roller (Side) (exercise), 154

Foam roller series, 99–104

Foam rollers (self-massage), 153–54

Football, exercise program, 45

Frontal Raises (exercise), 123

Frozen shoulder, 17–18; exercises, 52

G

Gentle and passive exercise series, 55–69

Glenohumeral (GH) joints, 6

Golf, exercise program 46

H

Hanging Arm Circles (exercise), 57

Hanging Dumbbell Squeeze (exercise), 147

Hockey, exercise program, 46

Horizontal Triceps Extension (exercise), 130

Humerus, 6

I

I's, Y's, and T's (exercise), 85–86; on Roller, 103–104. *See also* T's with Band; Y's with Band

Ice, 155

Immobilization, 26

Impingement, tendinitis. *See* Shoulder impingement

Inappropriate/controversial exercises, 36–39

Infraspinatus muscles, 9

Injuries: do's and don'ts, 35; prevention, 30–39; rehabilitation, 24–28; and repetitive motion, 12–13; types, 25. *See also specific injuries*

Instability. *See* shoulder instability

Internal Rotation (Door), 116

Internal Rotation (Side-Lying), 90

Internal Rotation Stretch (exercise), 67

Internal Rotation (Supine), 89

Internal Rotation with Band (exercise), 132

Internal rotations (exercises), 67, 89, 90, 116, 132

Isometric Frontal Lift (exercise), 119

Isometric Rear Lift (exercise), 120
Isometric Shoulder Blade Squeeze (exercise), 118

J
Joint capsules, 8
Joints, 6; illustrated, 7

L
Lateral Drops (exercise), 95
Lateral Raises (exercise), 124
Latissimus dorsi muscles, 9
Levator scapulae muscles, 9
Ligaments, 7

M
Massage. *See* Self-massage exercise series
Macro trauma, 25
Medical care, 5, 11. *See also specific conditions*
Micro trauma, 25
Mixed martial arts, exercise, program, 48
Muscles, 8–9; illustrated, 9

N
Neuropathways, 10

O
Office jobs, exercise program, 49
Over the Top (exercise), 66
Overuse tendinitis, 16

P
Passive and gentle exercise series, 55–69
Pec stretch (Basic) (exercise), 61
Pec stretches (exercises), 61, 121
Pectoralis major and minor muscles, 9
Pendulum (Across Body) (exercise), 56
Pendulum (Forward and Backward) (exercise), 55
Physiological variants, and shoulder dysfunction, 10
Picture Frame (exercise), 63
Pilates, Joseph, quoted, 30
Polymyalgia rheumatica, 15
Presses (exercises), 93, 97, 113, 136, 137, 145
Programs. *See* Exercise programs

Prone Crossing Guard (exercise), 148
Pull-Downs (exercise), 135
Pull-Overs (exercise), 94
Push Backs (exercise), 79
Push-ups (exercises), 92, 117

R
Raises (exercise), 123, 124
Range of motion exercise series, 70–81
Reaches (exercises), 64, 114
Rehabilitation, 24–28
Reinjuries, prevention, 30–39
Repetitive motion injuries, 12–13; exercises, 51
Reps, 43
Rescue Me (exercise), 77
Resistance bands. *See* Exercise bands
Resistance conditioning exercise series, 122–48
Reverse Fly with Band (exercise), 126
Reverse Lift (exercise), 96
Rhomboid major and minor muscles, 9
Roller exercise series, 99–104
Rotator Cuff (External Rotation) (exercise), 81
Rotator cuffs, 8; injuries, 16–17; exercises, 51; muscles, 8

S
Safety tips, 42. *See also* Injuries
Scapulas, 6
Scapulothoracic (ST) joints, 6
Seated Rowing (exercise), 134
Self-massage exercise series, 149–55
Serratus anterior muscles, 9
Serving Tray (exercise), 131
Shoulder abduction zones, 33-34
Shoulder Blade Pinch (exercise), 74
Shoulder Blade Push-Up (exercise), 92
Shoulder blades. *See* Scapulas
Shoulder Box (exercise), 58
Shoulder exercises. *See* Exercise programs
Shoulder Extension (Basic) (exercise), 125
Shoulder extension zones, 34
Shoulder extensions (exercises), 125, 142

Shoulder flexion zones, 34
Shoulder girdles, 6, 11
Shoulder impingement, 11–12, 16; exercises, 51
Shoulder instability, 14; exercises, 52
Shoulder Roll (exercise), 59
Shoulder Slaps (exercise), 102
Shoulders: anatomy, 6–9; exercises, 36–155; problems, 10–23; rehabilitation, 24–28
Shrug (Basic) (exercise), 141
Shrugs (exercises), 141, 146
Side Clock (exercise), 107
Softball, exercise program, 44
Soup can pours (exercises), 71, 143
Sports-related exercise programs, 44–48
Stabilizer muscles, 8–9
Stabilizers, static and dynamic, 9
Static Pec Stretch (exercise), 121
Sternoclavicular (SC) joints, 6
Sternums, 6
Stick Press (exercise), 97
Stick Up (exercise), 111
Stick/cane exercise series, 93–98
Straight-Arm Stretch (exercise), 84
Stretches. See specific exercises and programs
Subjective shoulder scale assessment, 11
Subluxation, 14; exercises, 52
Subscapularis muscles, 9
Supine Press (exercise), 93
Supraspinatus muscles, 9
Swimming, exercise program, 47
Sword Fighter (Basic) (exercise), 128
Sword Fighters (exercises), 127, 128

T
T's with Band (exercise), 139. See also I's, Y's, and T's

Table Reach (exercise), 64
Table Stretch (exercise), 69
Tendinitis, 11–16, 18–20; exercises, 52
Tendons, 7
Tennis, exercise program, 47
Tennis ball methods 149–52
Teres major and minor muscles, 9
Thoracic outlet region, 20
Thoracic Outlet Syndrome (TOS), 20–23
Touch Down (exercise), 78
Trapezius muscles, 9
Two-hour rule, 26, 54

U
Upper-Back Stretch (exercise), 72

V
Volleyball, exercise program 48

W
Wall Circles (exercise), 108
Wall/door exercise series, 105–21
Wall Push-Up (exercise), 117
Wall Reach (exercise), 114
Warm-ups, importance, 43, 52
The Wave (exercise), 73
Windmills on Roller (exercise), 100
Wood Chops (exercise), 75
Work-related exercise programs, 49
Wrestling, exercise program, 48

Y's with Band (exercise), 138. See also I's, Y's, and T's

The Zipper (exercise), 80
Zones, of shoulder movement, 33–34

OTHER BOOKS FROM KARL KNOPF

Healthy Hips Handbook: Exercises for Treating and Preventing Common Hip Joint Injuries
$14.95
Healthy Hips Handbook is designed to help prevent hip problems for some and, for those with existing hip problems, provide post-rehabilitation exercises.

Core Strength for 50+: A Customized Program for Safely Toning Ab, Back, and Oblique Muscles
$15.95
Core Strength for 50+ has everything you need to improve posture, enhance sports performance, guarantee lower-back health, and avoid injury.

Foam Roller Workbook: Illustrated Step-by-Step Guide to Stretching, Strengthening and Rehabilitative Techniques, 2nd edition
$15.95
Details a comprehensive program for using the foam roller to recover from injury, reverse everyday pain, and stay healthy in the future.

Kettlebells for 50+: Safe and Customized Programs for Building and Toning Every Muscle
$15.95
Provides sport-specific workouts that allow aging athletes to maintain the flexibility, strength, and speed needed to win.

Make the Pool Your Gym: No-Impact Water Workouts for Getting Fit, Building Strength, and Rehabbing from Injury
$14.95
Shows how to create an effective and efficient water workout that can build strength, improve cardiovascular fitness, and burn calories.

Stretching for 50+: A Customized Program for Increasing Flexibility, Avoiding Injury, and Enjoying an Active Lifestyle, 2nd edition
$15.95
This book shows the 50+ individual how to maintain and improve flexibility by incorporating stretching into one's life. Specially designed programs cater to every fitness level.

To order these books call 800-377-2542 or 510-601-8301, fax 510-601-8307, e-mail ulysses@ ulyssespress.com, or write to Ulysses Press, P.O. Box 3440, Berkeley, CA 94703. All retail orders are shipped free of charge. California residents must include sales tax. Allow two to three weeks for delivery.

ACKNOWLEDGMENTS

It is a joy to work with such a team of professionals, without whose skill and expertise this book would not have been possible. I would like to sincerely thank, Claire Chun and Renee Rutledge, whose attention to detail and ability to explain complex concepts in user-friendly terms is without parallel. Thanks also to models Samuel Harvell, Scott Mathison, Meredith Miller, Bernadett Otterbein, and Toni Silver for their patience, and to Austin Forbord and his team at Rapt Productions, who were able to capture the essence of the exercises so well. I'd like to thank acquisitions editor Keith Riegert for his vision. Lastly, a special note of appreciation to two people who served as my fact checkers: Dr. Fiona Gilbert and my son Chris Knopf.

ABOUT THE AUTHOR

Dr. Karl Knopf, or Dr. Karl, as his students used to call him, has been involved in the health and fitness of older adults and the disabled for over 40 years. During this time, he has worked in almost every aspect of the industry, from personal training and therapy to consultation. While at Foothill College, Karl was the coordinator of the Adaptive Fitness Technician Program and Life Long Learning Institute. He taught disabled students and undergraduates about corrective exercise. In addition to teaching, Karl developed the "Fitness Educators of Older Adults Association" to guide trainers of older adults. Currently Karl is a director at the International Sports Science Association and is on the advisor board of PBS's *Sit and Be Fit* show.

In his spare time, he has spoken at conferences, authored many articles, and written numerous books, including *Stretching for 50+*, *Make the Pool Your Gym*, *Resistance Band Workouts*, and *Beat Osteoporosis with Exercise*. He was a frequent guest on both radio and print media on issues pertaining to senior fitness and the disabled.